Headaches

Betty Ann Falletta

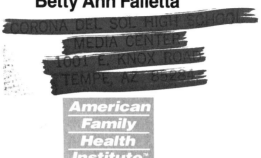

American Family Health Institute™

Medical Board

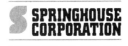

SPRINGHOUSE CORPORATION

SPRINGHOUSE, PA.

Program Director
Stanley Loeb

Clinical Director
Barbara McVan, RN

Art Director
John Hubbard

Editor
Richard Stull

Designers
Julie Carleton
Linda Franklin

Editorial Services Manager
David Moreau

Senior Production Manager
Deborah Meiris

Production Coordinator
Sally Johnson

The charter of the American Family Health Institute is to research and produce high-quality publications that enhance the health of individuals and their families. Essential to health are physical, emotional, and social well-being, not just the absence of illness or infirmity. The Institute's Medical Board has produced the *Health and Fitness* books to share up-to-date and authoritative information that can give readers greater personal control over their health maintenance.

Library of Congress Cataloging-in-Publication Data
Falletta, Betty Ann, 1940-
  Headaches.
  (Health & Fitness)
  Includes index.
  1. Headache—Popular works. I.
Dudrick, Stanley J. II. American Family
Health Institute. Medical Board. III. Title.
IV. Series: Health and fitness series. [DNLM:
1. Headache—popular works. WL 342 F195h]
RB128.F35 1986 616.07'2 86-5775
ISBN 0-87434-069-1

The procedures and explanations given in this publication are based on research and consultation with medical and nursing authorities. To the best of our knowledge, these procedures and explanations reflect currently accepted medical practice; nevertheless, they can't be considered absolute and universal recommendations. For individual application, treatment suggestions must be considered in light of the individual's health, subject to a doctor's specific recommendations. The authors and the publisher disclaim responsibility for any adverse effects resulting directly or indirectly from the suggested procedures, from any undetected errors, or from the reader's misunderstanding of the text.

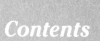

Contents

Headaches

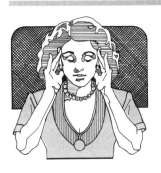

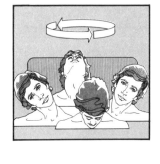

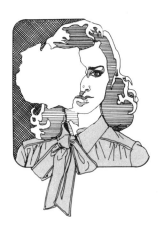

1

Understanding Symptoms

A symptom is evidence of a disorder or disease; it tells you that something is wrong. Most headaches are stress-related symptoms.

Headaches are probably our most common physical complaint because in one form or another they affect almost everyone. (Some studies indicate that over 90% of the population suffer occasional headaches.) Yet, the average headache sufferer knows little about how a headache causes pain or how the brain reacts to the pain.

This book discusses and explains the different types of headaches. Along the way, you'll learn how your body alerts you to pain. If you suffer occasional or chronic headaches, you'll learn ways that you may prevent them. You'll also learn ways to treat a headache without medication and how to decide when you need to see a doctor.

Symptom or disorder?

A symptom is evidence of a disorder or disease; it tells you that something is wrong. When you have one or more symptoms of a disorder or disease, you feel out of balance—not as well as you usually do. Pain, fever, nausea, dizziness, and chills are examples of symptoms, not diseases.

Sometimes, a condition that seems to be a symptom of a disorder or disease turns out to be a minor, temporary disorder that results from abusing your body in some way. For example, vomiting can be a symptom of intestinal tract blockage, stomach virus, or food poisoning, or it may be a temporary disorder caused by eating too fast or too much. Indigestion can be a symptom of stomach ulcers (a disorder), or it may result from overeating. Of course, you feel just as sick in either case, but learning to interpret your body's signals and being more aware of its needs are important keys in treating and preventing disorders and diseases that threaten your health.

Most headaches are symptoms

Most headaches are stress-related symptoms, not life-threatening disorders. A headache can be the symptom of infection, muscular tension, emotional problems, and, in rare instances, serious illness. Physical abuses as different as lack of sleep, alcohol overconsumption, or reading in awkward positions can result in headaches. Before you can effectively treat and prevent severe and frequent headaches, you must find out what they can tell you. Are your headaches symptoms of emotional stress? of physical stress? Do either of your parents suffer migraines? Did you injure your head recently? Do you get a headache every time you perform a particular activity? Do other symptoms accompany the headache pain? These are but a few of the questions you must try to answer before you look for treatments.

Headache: Disorder and symptom

Most physical complaints—pain, fever, and nausea, for example—are symptoms of an underlying disorder or disease. Sometimes, though, a complaint can be either a symptom or a disorder itself. Headache is one such complaint. A headache may be a temporary, minor disorder caused by such factors as fatigue, stress, or alcohol overconsumption, or it may be a symptom of a more serious problem.

Headache

may be a disorder

may be a symptom of an underlying disorder

- *muscle tension headache caused by fatigue, stress, or other factors*
- *vascular headache caused by drug or alcohol use, for example*
- *migraine headache (cause unknown)*

- *infection*
- *high blood pressure*
- *brain tumor or disease*
- *head injury*
- *disorders of the eyes, teeth, ears, or sinuses*
- *psychological or emotional problems*

2

How You Feel Pain

If you are worried, anxious, frightened, depressed, fatigued, overworked, or discontented, you may feel pain more acutely than you otherwise would.

Pain is a complex phenomenon. By definition, it's unpleasant and inseparable from the person experiencing it. But pain differs from person to person. Two people with the same injury don't necessarily feel the same pain sensations. You may also react differently to similarly caused pain at different times. The way you respond to pain depends on many factors—psychological, physiologic, social, and cultural. If you are worried, anxious, frightened, depressed, fatigued, overworked, or discontented, you may feel pain more acutely than you otherwise would. Emotions don't cause the pain, but they can intensify your reaction to it.

Your religious beliefs, the way family members reacted to your pain or to their own when you were growing up, the physical surroundings in which you experience pain, and even your social status can affect the way you respond. The nature of a disorder or disease that may cause pain can greatly affect how you experience the discomfort. For example, someone responding to the seemingly pointless pain of a migraine may suffer more acutely than a person experiencing the pain following cosmetic surgery or childbirth.

Pain threshold

The point at which you begin to feel pain when nerve endings are stimulated is called your pain threshold. No matter what your upbringing or your genetic makeup, most people perceive pain at about the same point of stimulation. For example, everyone's skin will burn or freeze at specific temperatures; however, whether you choose to acknowledge the pain of heat or cold is another matter. You may learn to increase your tolerance for pain or raise your pain threshold, but you can't lower your pain threshold.

How pain messages reach the brain

A pain message may originate in an injured body part. If you strike your finger with a hammer, your finger will immediately hurt where the hammer struck. Your body will quickly release both pain-inducing and pain-sensitizing chemicals in the nerve endings close to the injury point. These released chemicals

Endorphins

Your body produces chemicals that regulate pain. Among these are endorphins, made by the pituitary and hypothalamus glands. Endorphins block pain or alter your perception of it. Many activities, such as vigorous exercise, stimulate endorphin production.

don't all have the same function. Prostaglandins, for example, cause swelling and inflammation so that circulation to the area increases and infection-fighting blood cells gather.

Fluids within nerve fibers enable nerves to generate electric impulses that carry the pain message from one nerve to the next. A pain impulse travels along the length of a nerve until it reaches the junction between two nerves, known as the synapse. There, chemical transmitters move the message across the gap between the nerves.

The pain message continues to travel to the dorsal horn of the spinal cord. From there, it travels to the thalamus, making you aware of the pain sensation. How the pain message travels from the thalamus to the brain's cerebral cortex, where you register the location and intensity of the pain, remains the least understood part of this process.

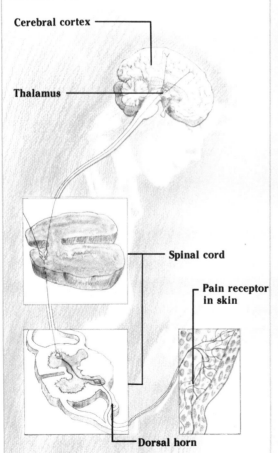

Cerebral cortex

Thalamus

Spinal cord

Pain receptor in skin

Dorsal horn

The pain process

• *A pain message begins at the nerve ending in the injured body part.*

• *In response to the pain message, the body releases chemicals that change the pain message to an electric impulse.*

• *The impulse then travels to the dorsal horn of the spinal cord.*

• *The impulse reaches the brain's sensory center, the thalamus. At this point, you become conscious of the pain.*

• *The impulse travels to the brain's cerebral cortex, which records the pain's location and intensity.*

8

Quick response: Pain reflex arc

- *A painful stimulus starts at the sensory neuron.*
- *This impulse travels to the dorsal horn and into the spinal cord.*
- *The pain impulse passes through the spinal cord to the brain.*
- *The motor response doesn't wait for brain processing. Instead, the interneuron passes the impulse to the motor neuron, which causes a reflex action.*

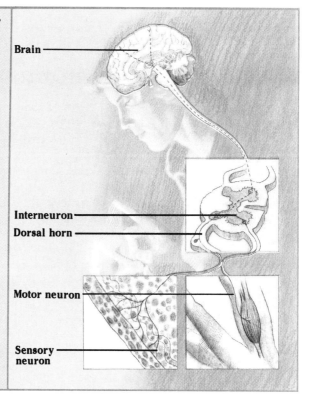

Brain

Interneuron

Dorsal horn

Motor neuron

Sensory neuron

The nervous system

The nervous system, your body's highly developed communication network, receives and transmits messages throughout your body. It receives information about the outside world and relays this information to the cells and tissues in your body's organs, enabling you to adapt to external events. The nervous system also records and responds to stimuli within the body.

The brain and nerves together make up the nervous system. The brain and spinal column constitute the central nervous system (CNS). Nerves that relay messages to and from the central nervous system are part of the peripheral nervous system (PNS).

Two major cell types that make up the nervous system are neuroglial cells and neurons. Neuroglial cells don't transmit or receive messages; they supply neurons with food and energy. (After an injury to the central nervous system, neuroglial cells may reproduce rapidly. Some CNS tumors result from overgrowth of neuroglial cells.) Neurons are classifed into two types: sensory (afferent) neurons and motor (efferent) neurons. Both sensory and motor neurons transmit impulses from the central nervous system

Central vs. peripheral nervous system

Your central nervous system (CNS) consists of your brain and spinal cord (shaded below). This core serves as your nervous control center. Your peripheral nervous system links your CNS with the rest of your body.

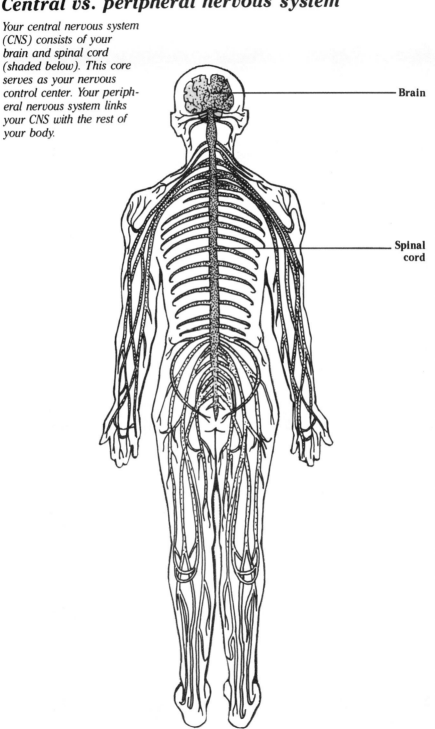

Brain

Spinal
cord

Nerve cell

Nerve cells are basic pieces in the pain process. A nerve cell, or neuron, consists of the cell body and long branches (axons) stretching from both ends. The axons, the main conducting fibers, and their terminals, the dendrites, spread throughout the body. The neuron's cell body is housed within the brain or spinal cord.

Neuron bundles make up your nerves. The thick bundle of nerves running from your brain's base down your back is your spinal column.

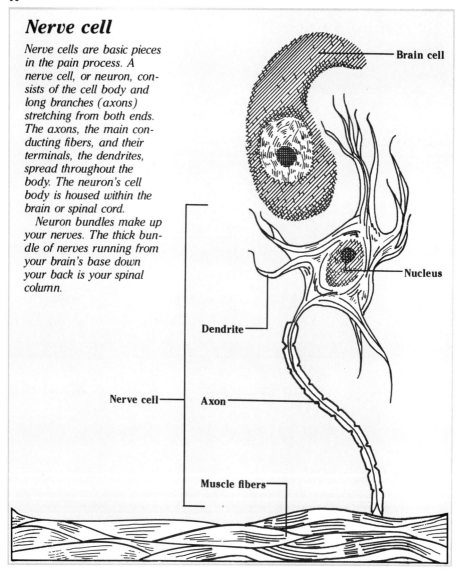

to other tissues. Sensory nerves, however, relay sensory messages (sight, sound, taste, smell, touch), whereas motor nerves control body movements.

Neurons are housed within the brain and spinal cord. The axons, the main conducting fibers, and their terminals, the dendrites, spread throughout the body.

By working together, the central nervous system and the peripheral nervous system create a communication network by which sensory messages are received, interpreted, and sent. The peripheral nervous system picks up pain messages, and the central nervous system interprets them. The peripheral ner-

Afferent–Efferent: What's the difference?

Think of afferent nerves as passageways for impulses away from an injured area: They carry messages from the peripheral nervous system (PNS) to the central nervous system (CNS). Efferent nerves carry messages from the CNS to the PNS.

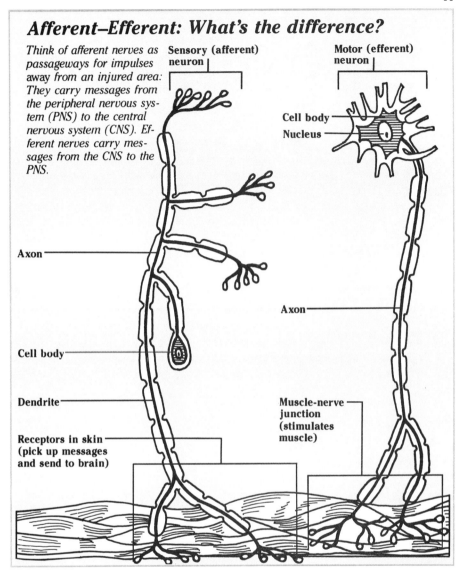

Sensory (afferent) neuron

Motor (efferent) neuron

Cell body
Nucleus

Axon

Cell body

Dendrite

Receptors in skin (pick up messages and send to brain)

Axon

Muscle-nerve junction (stimulates muscle)

vous system consists of 31 pairs of spinal nerves that connect the spinal cord with various body parts. Peripheral nerves are made up of bundles of nerve fibers bound together with sheaths of connective tissue.

Different nerves in the peripheral nervous system have different functions. Motor (efferent) peripheral nerves may contain fibers that convey messages from the brain and spinal cord to the muscles in the head, trunk, and limbs. Sensory (afferent) peripheral nerves carry messages from the brain to the sense organs of touch, sight, sound, taste, or smell. Many peripheral nerves contain both motor and sensory fibers.

3

What Hurts When Your Head Aches

Most headache pain isn't from aching brain tissue, though enlarged blood vessels will actually make your tissues hurt.

Probably you assume that your brain tissue hurts when you have a headache. In fact, though, your brain tissue usually doesn't feel the sensations you describe when you have a headache. Yet part of your brain interprets pain messages. You become conscious of pain when the thalamus, a sensory center deep inside the brain, receives a message from the spinal cord. The pain message then travels to the cortex, the brain's outer layer of nerve cells, which notes the pain's location and intensity.

Brain

Some headache pain can be in your brain, though. Pain can result from overstretched or narrowed blood vessels there. Pressure from inflamed tissue and from tissue growth can also cause pain. Besides blood vessel pain, you can also experience pain in the membranes surrounding the brain and spinal column (the meninges).

Bones

Your skull's bones don't feel pain even when they're injured; however, headaches can result from skull injuries that press on the pain-sensitive parts of the meninges or from inflamed tissue that squeezes sensitive nerve endings and blood vessels. The eye sockets and other skull openings contain pain-sensitive nerves and blood vessels. The bone formations that shape your face also create about 20 air cavities lined with mucus-secreting cells. These air cavities, or sinuses, cause pain when they become infected and inflamed and when abnormal tissue growth within these spaces presses on other tissue.

Your backbone and neck protect and support your spinal column. Upper back and neck injuries can irritate pain-sensitive parts of the meninges, force muscles to contract, or press on nerve endings and blood vessels, leading to headache.

Muscles, blood vessels, and nerves

All tissue outside the skull, especially arteries, can cause pain. When any of the layers of overlapping muscles covering the head bones and neck become inflamed from strain or other injury, you may have

Cross section of the spinal cord

The spinal cord, the bridge between a pain impulse and the brain, consists of gray matter surrounded by white matter. The gray matter includes the ventral (anterior) and dorsal (posterior) horns. Different types of nerve fibers enter different horns. A segment of each dorsal horn, the substantia gelatinosa, is important in regulating pain impulses.

In the white matter that surrounds the gray matter, many nerve fiber tracts relay messages to and from the brain.

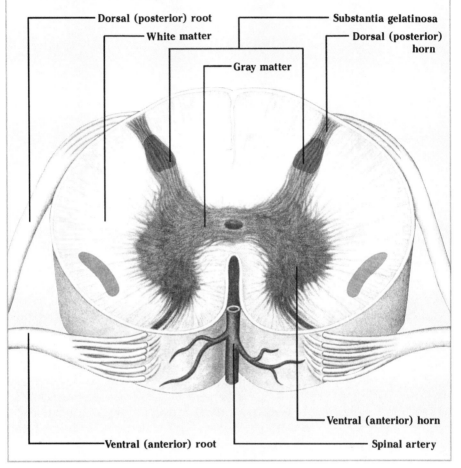

Dorsal (posterior) root
White matter
Gray matter
Substantia gelatinosa
Dorsal (posterior) horn
Ventral (anterior) horn
Ventral (anterior) root
Spinal artery

pain. The blood vessels and nerves within the overlapping muscle layers enable the muscles to feel pain. Stretched blood vessels can cause throbbing pain because the nerves and muscles responsible for the shrinking and expanding of blood vessels may not work properly. During prolonged contraction, muscles press on pain-sensitive nerves and blood vessels.

The cranial nerves that carry messages between the brain stem and different parts of the head and face, especially the eyes and mouth, are often involved in headaches.

4

Vascular Headaches: The Migraines

Blood vessels within and around the skull (cranium) change during many types of headaches, but no one knows for certain how or why these changes occur. Despite the controversy about the reasons for these blood vessel changes, most experts agree that some headaches involve abnormal blood vessel narrowing (constriction) and expansion (dilation). Headaches that involve blood vessel narrowing and expansion are called vascular headaches. The three major types of vascular headaches include classic migraine, common migraine, and cluster headaches.

Key points about migraines

—For the most part, migraines are a familial disorder. If either of your parents had migraines, you may be a migraine sufferer.

—Migraine is not a disease.

—Some students of migraines have tried to describe a "migraine personality," but no one has succeeded.

—Migraine headaches are more painful than other headache types.

—Between 10% and 20% of migraine sufferers have classic migraines. The rest have common migraines.

—More women suffer from classic and common migraines, whereas more men suffer from cluster headaches. The figures, however, may not tell the true story since fewer men than women seek medical help for their problems.

—Infants, children, and adolescents suffer migraines, but adults in their twenties and older experience greater migraine pain.

—While migraines are difficult to diagnose, the patient can help the doctor by providing a detailed medical and family history and by keeping a headache diary.

—Migraines may be prevented, but they can't be cured.

Classic and common migraines

A migraine is not simply a severe vascular headache. Migraine ailments are accompanied by a wide variety of associated discomforts, some of which may seem to have very little to do with head pain. Common

No self-diagnosis
Because you may easily misunderstand the complex migraine syndrome, you should not try to diagnose yourself. If you identify with the syndromes you read about in this book, you should consult your doctor. Only he can prescribe the medications you may need. Furthermore, you should not take any medication without giving a medical history and having a physical examination.

Changes in the brain's blood vessels

This model of the brain's blood vessels shows how complex and intricate a system it is.

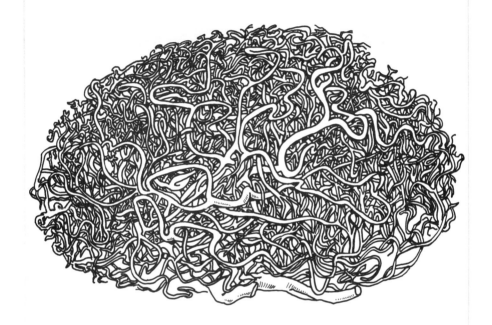

Changes in the width of these blood vessels can affect the brain cells. For example, enlarged blood vessels press the brain cells together, putting pressure on brain tissue and causing pain.

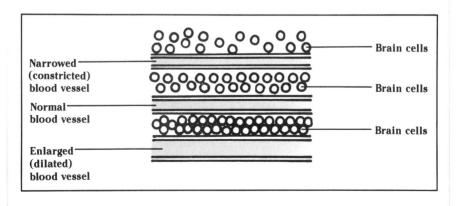

Brain cells

Narrowed (constricted) blood vessel

Brain cells

Normal blood vessel

Brain cells

Enlarged (dilated) blood vessel

Symptoms of migraine headaches

Classic and common migraine headaches differ, but they share some symptoms. Here are the details.

Classic migraine

• Preheadache symptoms include visual disturbances such as bright lights and zigzag lines, sensory disturbances (tingling of hands, face, or lips), motor disturbances, possible weight gain, muscle soreness, fever, cold hands or feet, sweating, paleness, and confusion.
• Recurrent and periodic headaches about ½ hour after the prodrome.
• Headache that usually begins as one-sided.
• Typical headache phase symptoms include nausea, diarrhea or vomiting, nasal stuffiness, paleness, abdominal pains, aversion to light or noise, and total body achiness.

Common migraine

• Typical preheadache symptoms include irritability, fatigue, weight gain, and sudden mood change.
• Headache that usually begins as one-sided.
• Typical headache phase symptoms include nasal stuffiness, nausea, diarrhea or constipation, paleness, abdominal pains, and aversion to light or noise.

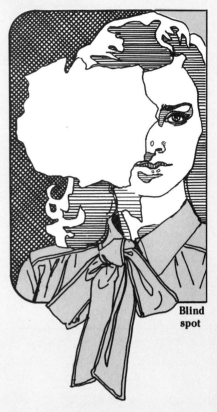

Blind
spot

Three visual distortions that forewarn of classic migraine

discomforts may involve the eyes, nose, stomach, intestines, and bladder. Yet these discomforts vary among people who suffer different types of migraines and among people who have the same type of migraine.

Preheadache phase. The classic migraine sufferer has what's called an aura, or prodrome—symptoms that precede the headache. These symptoms distinguish the classic migraine from other migraine types. The aura is often painless but distracting, and it may last from about 15 minutes to more than an hour. The most common preheadache symptoms include visual disturbances such as flashbulb-like blind spots, zigzag lines, visual distortions, and tunnel vision. Other symptoms include tingling or numbness on one side of the body, increased skin sensitivity, motor disturbances such as staggering gait and slurred

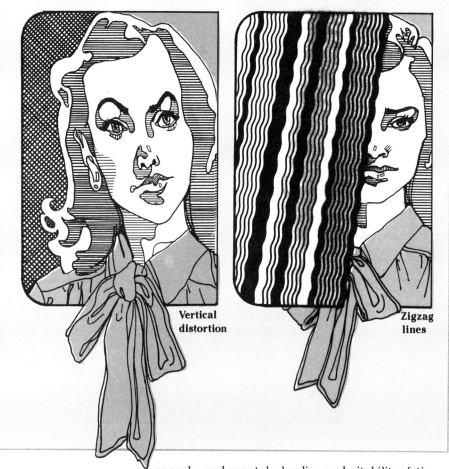

Vertical distortion

Zigzag lines

speech, and mental cloudiness. Irritability, fatigue, fever, sweating, paleness, confusion, and cold hands or feet may also characterize the aura.

Although the well-defined aura of the classic migraine does not precede the common migraine, many common migraine sufferers report nonspecific symptoms before the headache. They claim that they can predict an oncoming migraine by such symptoms as weight gain, irritability, sudden mood change, and mental fuzziness.

The headache phase. Both the classic and common migraine have essentially the same headache phase. For the classic migraine sufferer, the headache will begin about ½ hour after the prodrome. For both the classic and common migraine sufferer, the headache usually begins as a throbbing pain on one side of the head. (In fact, the word "migraine" is derived from a

Identifying your headache

You may be a migraine sufferer if your headaches:
- *occur on one side of your head*
- *recur in patterns*
- *are associated with irritability, nausea and vomiting, diarrhea, chills, paleness, sweating, or sensitivity or aversion to light (photophobia).*

Greek word meaning "half head.")

The pain may then settle into one location or move about from the forehead to one side of the head, to the top of the head, to the eyes, or to both temples. Sometimes, the pain spreads to the jaw or one nostril. At times, the scalp, face, and neck may be tender to the touch. In this stage of the migraine, sufferers usually complain of nausea or vomiting. Luckily for some, vomiting relieves the pain. Other symptoms may include total body achiness, chills and feverlike symptoms, a great sensitivity to light or noise, paleness, puffiness, nasal stuffiness, abdominal pain, diarrhea, or constipation.

Before the classic or common migraine headache begins, the body retains water and salt. Toward the end of the headache phase, the sufferer may urinate frequently. In this way, the body gets rid of the excessive salt and water. Although the 1-hour or the more-than-a-day migraine attack does eventually end, a migraine leaves aftereffects. The sufferer may have sore muscles, feel totally exhausted, and experience mental fuzziness for some time.

Who gets migraines

If your parents or other family members suffer migraine headaches, you may become a migraine sufferer. Migraines often first appear between a person's adolescence and early twenties, but they may develop before and after this age range, too. Some individuals develop nonheadache symptoms several years before they experience actual headaches. Recurrent vomiting in anxious children, stomachaches, and motion sickness are among the symptoms that could signal migraines at a later time.

Treatment: Migraine first aid

Migraine headaches are temporary. If you did nothing to treat a migraine attack, it would eventually disappear. Fortunately, you don't have to suffer the migraine discomfort, especially when the episodes are frequent or predictable. Try one or more of the following treatments to diminish your discomfort.

—Don't ignore the migraine. Stop what you're doing. Your head hurts because of expanded or swollen blood vessels, and the swelling will subside if you can relax. Go to a quiet room, turn off the lights, and lie down with your head slightly elevated. Breathe deeply and concentrate on relaxing.

—Drink a cup of coffee at the first sign of the migraine.

Using a cold pack

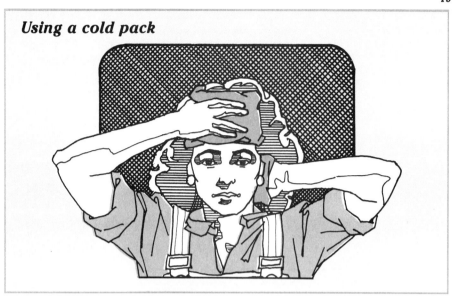

(Coffee shrinks swollen blood vessels.)
—Take two aspirin tablets or aspirin-substitute tablets if you can't tolerate aspirin.
—Apply a cold pack—a gel encased in plastic that can be kept in the freezer or refrigerator—or a cold washcloth to both your head and your neck. The cold may contract the enlarged blood vessels.
—Take a cold shower or cold bath.
—Apply pressure to your temples. Locate the bony ridge between your eye's outer corner and your eyebrow's outer end. Move your index finger toward your ear until you find a small hollow. Using your left-hand index finger on your left temple and your right-hand

Applying pressure to your temples

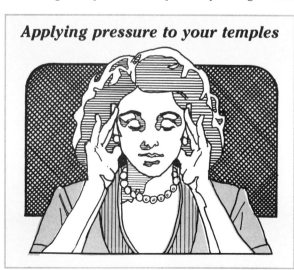

Two painkillers
Narcotics and aspirin act on two different levels of the nervous system. Narcotics act mainly on the central nervous system (the brain and spinal column). Aspirin acts on the peripheral nervous system (the nerves that branch out from the central nervous system to the rest of the body).

Case study: Classic migraine

Eleanor Miller, age 30, changed jobs after 10 years with the same firm. Eleanor's headaches apparently started about the time of her move. She complained of nasal stuffiness that became worse during the spring and fall. Then she noticed a pattern to her headaches. About the same time each month, 2 days before her period, Eleanor experienced a throbbing pain in her left temple, and her migraine came on for at least 2 days.

Before the headache pain started, she experienced light-headedness, a tingling sensation in her upper arm, and blurry vision. Eleanor suffered classic migraine headaches.

index finger on your right temple, press the area as you count to 10. Then repeat. (For further details, see "Acupuncture and acupressure," pages 47 to 50.)

Treatment: Migraine medication
—Ergotamine (Cafergot tablets or suppositories, Medihaler Ergotamine, Ergomar, Ergostat), alone or in combination with caffeine, is the prescription medication that most doctors recommend for a migraine attack. The drug has a unique property: it works for migraine headaches but not for other headaches. Ergotamine is a powerful vasoconstrictor; that is, it can greatly reduce the swelling in vessels. Ergotamine comes in many different combination prescriptions: ergotamine with caffeine, sedatives, barbiturates, or belladonna (Cafergot P-B, Wigraine, Bellergal) to relax the intestines. Your ergotamine prescription will depend on your symptoms and your doctor's diagnosis.

Ergotamine can effectively stop a migraine if you take it at the first sign of attack. For the classic migraine, take the medication during the prodrome—the preheadache phase. If your migraines make you vomit, you can't take your medicine orally, so your doctor may prescribe ergotamine as a suppository. For the common migraine, take the medication when the pain begins.

—Tranquilizers, sedatives, antidepressants, and narcotic painkillers (codeine combined with aspirin or

Narcotics
Codeine, morphine, and heroin are narcotics. Narcotics originally came from a flower called the opium poppy, and the drugs were called opiates. Today, drugs similar to opiates are produced in the laboratory.

aspirin substitute) may help migraine sufferers who don't respond to ergotamine or can't take the drug.
—Indomethacin (Indocin) and over-the-counter ibuprofen (Advil, Nuprin) are anti-inflammatory pain relievers. In addition, they inhibit the secretion of certain body chemicals (prostaglandins) that cause blood vessels to expand and blood to clot, which are associated with the migraine syndrome.

Migraine triggers

Before you and your doctor can effectively diagnose and treat your migraines, you must identify what triggers the attacks. Triggers and causes, however, are not the same. A migraine trigger refers to provoking psychological or physical factors that may set off the migraine. Migraine triggers could include such things as an argument with a co-worker or lack of sleep.

By contrast, the causes of a migraine are complex biochemical and physiologic reactions. The inherited tendency, or your genetic makeup, causes the migraine syndrome. The trigger sets off the attack.

Some of your migraine triggers will be obvious to you, but others will be difficult to identify. Identifying your triggers may require a little medical detective work on your part.

Allergies. Anyone can have allergies, including migraine sufferers. In fact, the symptoms of allergies and migraines are similar, and both disorders raise the body's histamine level. (Histamines, substances that occur in all animal and vegetable tissue, can

Mixed headache
If you have a migraine headache, you may hold your head in a rigid way, and the awkward posture may set off an additional muscle contraction (tension) headache.

For more information
If you have any questions about the testing of over-the-counter or prescription drugs, write to the Food and Drug Administration for brochures:
Food and Drug Administration
5600 Fishers Lane
Rockville, MD 20852

Migraine triggers and causes

Simply stated, a migraine trigger is any physical or psychological factor that sets off a migraine headache. Although your genes and other things may make you susceptible to these headaches, the migraine's actual cause is your body's response to the trigger.

Trigger
A certain food, beverage, or drug; too much or too little sleep; an argument; stress; or another factor

Cause
Blood vessel narrowing and expansion in and around the skull

Result
Migraine headache

make your blood vessels swell; they also stimulate stomach juices.) Therefore, you might expect that antihistamines would help migraine as well as allergy sufferers; but, paradoxically, while antihistamines do help allergy sufferers, they don't help migraine sufferers.

Foods and drugs. The foods, beverages, chemical preservatives, and medications that you ingest can affect your migraine headaches. Cheese, chocolate, citrus fruit (especially oranges), meat, seafood, fatty food, and food containing monosodium glutamate (MSG) and nitrites (the preservative in hot dogs and other cured meats) are probably the most serious offenders. Chinese food, instant and canned soup, tenderizers and seasonings, instant gravies, and some TV dinners may contain large amounts of MSG.

Fasting, skipping meals, or going without food for over 5 or 6 hours can trigger a headache. If your migraines come on during the night, try eating a low-carbohydrate snack, such as a piece of chicken, some broiled fish, or green vegetables, at bedtime.

While caffeine narrows blood vessels, it stimulates the brain and heart and increases urine production. Excessive caffeine intake through coffee, tea, chocolate, cola drinks, over-the-counter headache and so-called sinus medications (Anacin, Excedrin, Vanquish, and Dristan, for example), and migraine medication (Cafergot) can cause mood and sleep disturbances, headaches, and withdrawal symptoms. But cutting back on the caffeine you're used to can also cause headaches.

Hormones and hormonal changes. For many women, the hormonal changes that occur in menstruation, pregnancy, menopause, and the taking of birth control pills or other hormones directly relate to migraine headaches. Mounting medical evidence indicates that women who are prone to migraines should not take birth control pills or estrogen compounds at menopause. You should consult your doctor about migraines associated with menstruation, hormonal medication, pregnancy, or menopause.

Hypertension. Hypertension, or high blood pressure, rarely causes headaches. When high blood pressure does cause a headache, it may be a very slight one that the victim experiences upon awakening. The migraine sufferer with high blood pressure, however,

Guidelines for taking prescription medication
DO:
• *Read labels and directions on prescriptions.*
• *Drink an 8-ounce glass of water when you take a pill.*
• *Call your doctor if you have any unusual side effects.*
• *Take medication only as directed.*
• *Keep drugs in a child-proof container or out of a child's reach.*
DON'T:
• *Take more than the prescribed dose.*
• *Take pills without drinking sufficient water.*
• *Give someone else your prescription pills.*
• *Leave prescription drugs where children can find them.*

Other stress triggers
For some people, glaring lights such as those you might see in oncoming night traffic, weather changes, the letdown of a weekend after a full week's work, and sexual intercourse can act as migraine triggers.

may have more frequent migraine attacks. Therefore, migraine sufferers need to have their blood pressure checked at least once a year.

Physical stress. Physical stress can trigger migraine headaches, with variations from person to person. Examples of stress triggers include:
—too much or too little sleep
—overexertion
—exercise if you aren't fit
—fatigue
—extremes of light, heat, cold, sound, or motion
—strong odors
—poor ventilation
—steam from cooking
—steam baths or saunas
—ill-fitting dentures, misalignment of teeth and the jaw (See *TMJ syndrome headache,* page 39.)
—extreme hunger
—a mild blow to the head.

Emotional stress. Emotional stress can provoke muscle contraction (tension) headaches, but the same kind of stress can also trigger migraine headaches. In many cases, emotional stress can trigger a mixed headache—a combination tension and migraine headache.

The end of stress can also trigger migraines. The sudden shift from stress to relaxation probably brings about the attack in the same way that a happy surprise and excitement can serve as migraine triggers.

Prevention: Migraine headaches
Some migraine sufferers can predict their attacks because they occur with such regularity. For example, women who get migraines before or at the beginning of each menstrual cycle usually know to expect an attack. Most migraine episodes, however, remain unpredictable.

If your migraines are either predictable or so frequent that they interfere with your life-style, you may be an excellent candidate for some of the new preventive measures. Of course, both the treatment and the prevention require medical assistance.

Preventive medications
—Your doctor may prescribe propranolol (Inderal), 160 to 240 mg daily, as a useful agent in migraine prevention. Among its many useful properties, propranolol prevents swelling of the arteries. This drug

How to prevent migraines without medication

- *Don't sleep late, even on your days off.*
- *Avoid abrupt climate changes.*
- *If you smoke, try to quit. Nicotine expands blood vessels, which can trigger migraines.*
- *Find out if medications you take for other conditions trigger your migraines. List all of them, and avoid any drugs that give you a migraine.*
- *Exercise regularly.*
- *If you don't know how to relax, learn. Take a yoga class, or learn how to meditate.*
- *If you get early morning migraines, eat a low-carbohydrate snack before bedtime.*
- *Either too little or too much caffeine can produce headaches, so pay attention to your intake.*

Daily or migraine headache?

Daily headaches aren't migraines; they're usually tension headaches. One common daily headache cause is ergotamine poisoning. You should use ergotamine daily only as a preventive drug for treating cluster headaches.

also causes a decrease in prostaglandins. Fewer prostaglandins reduces your blood's tendency to clot. According to headache researchers, prostaglandins and a blood clotting tendency are significant migraine triggers.

Migraine sufferers with asthma, lung disease, chronic heart failure, or diabetes, and those who take insulin, oral medication for hypoglycemia, or antidepressants should not take propranolol. On the other hand, migraine sufferers who can't tolerate ergotamine because of high blood pressure or angina pectoris (chest pain) may find propranolol very helpful. The drug helps prevent migraines while also lowering blood pressure and treating the angina.

—When other preventive measures have failed, your doctor may prescribe methysergide (Sansert), usually 4 to 8 mg daily. The drug acts paradoxically. First, it blocks the inflammatory and vasoconstrictor effects of serotonin, and then it helps the action of serotonin.

Migraine sufferers who are pregnant and those who have a peptic ulcer, peripheral vascular disease, or coronary artery disease should not take methysergide. Other side effects that may prevent its continued use include nausea, vomiting, gastrointestinal pain, diarrhea, dizziness, anxiety, or hallucinations.

—Clonidine (Catapres) is an antihypertensive (blood pressure–lowering) drug that may be useful in preventing migraines for those sensitive to foods containing tyramine—cheese, ripe bananas, red wine, nuts, chocolate, and sour cream, among others.

However, doctors use clonidine less frequently than propranolol (Inderal). The starting clonidine dosage is usually 0.1 to 0.15 mg daily. The consequences can be fatal if you suddenly discontinue the drug. Clonidine's side effects include mild gastrointestinal distress, weight gain, dry mouth, and drowsiness.

—Pizotifen is an antiserotonin agent that isn't yet available in the United States but is available in Canada and Europe. Recent emphasis on serotonin as a migraine cause has led to the introduction of antiserotonin drugs for migraine prevention (see page 26). A woman can't use antiserotonin during pregnancy. Its side effects include drowsiness, weight gain, and fatigue.

—While aspirin may not stop a migraine in progress, it may help prevent migraines if you take it in therapeutic doses. Don't take extra aspirin unless your doctor tells you to do so.

How aspirin prevents clotting

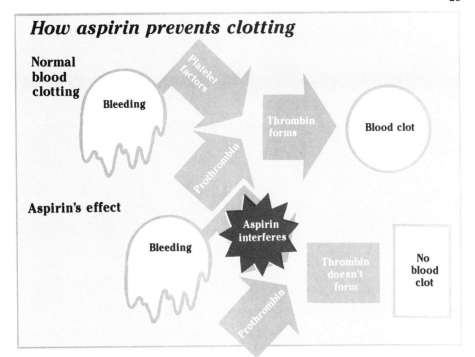

Normal blood clotting

Bleeding → Platelet factors → Thrombin forms → Blood clot

Prothrombin

Aspirin's effect

Bleeding → Aspirin interferes

Prothrombin → Thrombin doesn't form → No blood clot

What aspirin does
- It lowers fever.
- It reduces swelling.
- It relieves pain.

Rules for taking aspirin
- Follow the directions on the label. Don't exceed the recommended dosage.
- Call a doctor and discontinue aspirin if you have unusual side effects, including stomach pain, blood in urine or stool, nausea, or a ringing in your ears.
- Repeated headaches are a warning. Don't take aspirin for longer than a few days. The presence of aspirin in the bloodstream may make the diagnosis of chronic pain more difficult.
- Aspirin can be toxic. If you have small children in the house, keep aspirin out of a child's reach and in a childproof container.

Aspirin's anticlotting action helps to prevent platelet stickiness—important because of the correlation between classic migraine and strokes and heart attacks. Platelets play an important role in clotting, and some headache researchers have found that the platelets of migraine sufferers have an increased propensity to form clots, suggesting that this abnormality is responsible for strokes that complicate some migraines. Aspirin acts to stop the platelet action, thus reducing the risk of heart attack and stroke as well as preventing migraines.

Other anticlotting drugs called platelet antagonists include sulfinpyrazone (Anturane) and dipyridamole (Persantine).

—Doctors use calcium channel blockers (verapamil, nimodipine, nifedipine) extensively for treating heart conditions such as hypertension, angina pectoris, and irregular heartbeat (dysrhythmias). Calcium channel blockers prevent blood vessel narrowing by stopping calcium ion movement in the cells of the blood vessels. The effects of calcium channel blockers on different headache types are very promising. In tested subjects, 85% of vascular headache sufferers reported improvement, and classic migraine subjects reported that prodromes were either reduced or prevented. The FDA has yet to approve calcium channel blockers for migraine prevention.

Natural chemicals and headaches

Where amines come from
The following amines are found in food and can affect your blood vessels:
- dopamine (in fava beans)
- histamine (in some cheeses and in alcoholic beverages)
- octopamine (in some citrus fruits)
- tyramine (in red wine, aged cheeses, nuts, ripe bananas, beer)
- beta-phenylethylamine (in chocolate).

Two other amines come from your adrenal glands: epinephrine (adrenalin) and norepinephrine (noradrenalin). They also affect your blood vessels.

A migraine sufferer may overreact to concentrated amounts of certain chemical compounds, such as amines, that he eats or that the body makes. These chemicals influence behavior and moods and may cause the narrowing and widening of blood vessels. To understand some of the treatment and preventive medications for migraine and other headaches, you should become familiar with a few body chemicals that are the focus of much current headache research.

Amines form the basis of organic chemistry. They are natural nitrogen compounds. The body manufactures some amines; it removes others from food. And many headache researchers believe that the consumption of food and beverages containing too many amines can trigger migraines.

In concentrated amounts, amines can change the size of blood vessels. Blood pressure control, heart rate, brain activity, and nerve function are a few body functions affected by amines. If your body contains insufficient or overabundant amines, you may have neurologic or psychological problems. At least eight amines affect the expansion and narrowing of blood vessels.

Serotonin, a body-made amine, is stored in the blood in disk-shaped objects called platelets. High levels of serotonin increase stomach and intestinal activity and water retention. Some headache researchers claim that a high serotonin level in the migraine preheadache phase causes swelling of hands and feet and diarrhea. During the headache phase of a migraine attack, serotonin levels drop and some sufferers urinate frequently.

Platelets are important for blood clotting. When a blood vessel wall sustains an injury, blood platelets clump together near the injury site to narrow the blood vessel and prevent

Foods with tyramines

These foods contain enough tyramine to trigger your headaches:

Meat and fish
*Liver
Pickled herring
Dried sausage (including salami and pepperoni)
Smoked meat or fish*

Dairy products
Cheese (cottage and cream cheese are acceptable)

Beverages
*Beer
Wine (especially red wine)
Coffee (excessive amounts)*

Others
Chocolate

blood loss. Blood platelets in migraine sufferers readily clump together, which may account for the visual and speech disturbances in the pre-headache phase.

Tyramine, derived from the Greek word for cheese, is one of the many amines found in food. (See *Foods with tyramines* for more information.) Tyramine-rich foods can trigger migraines and alter blood vessels. Once inside the body, tyramines are broken down by monoamine oxidase (MAO). However, if you're taking an antidepressant that contains MAO inhibitors, you may suffer from headaches when you eat amine-rich food. Why? Because the MAO inhibitors prevent the breakdown of tyramines. Then the tyramines accumulate, causing headaches and possibly leading to high blood pressure and stroke.

Bradykinin, a chemical irritant, may lower your pain threshold. It's produced by the body at an inflammation site. For example, the fluid beneath a blister contains bradykinin. If the fluid were injected into another person, that person would experience severe pain. The chemical content of bradykinin resembles wasp venom.

Prostaglandins are chemicals found in all areas and organs of our bodies. Not all prostaglandins have been identified, but the 15 or more that have been identified have letter names with subscripts. PGA and PGE prostaglandins enlarge vessels. PGE_1 inhibits platelet grouping (blood clotting), whereas PGE_2 stimulates platelet grouping. PGA_2 and PGE_2 help regulate blood pressure. PGE_2 and PGE-alpha work during an inflammation. (Aspirin reaching an inflammation prevents damaged cells from giving off prostaglandins; and without the sensitizing effect of prostaglandins, the nerve endings don't react.)

What the serotonin facts may mean

Fact	Possible conclusion
Serotonin acts as a constricting agent in arteries and other blood vessels.	Serotonin plays a role in the early migraine attack phase when arteries narrow.
Blood serotonin levels rise when you vomit.	The increased serotonin level and its artery-constricting action account for the headache relief of some migraine sufferers after vomiting.
Serotonin prevents water excretion.	The high serotonin level in the preheadache phase accounts for the swelling of hands and feet of migraine sufferers.
The serotonin level is abnormally high in the migraine's preheadache phase.	The high serotonin level causes blood vessel narrowing in the preheadache phase.
An injection of serotonin relieves migraine headache.	Serotonin's ability to narrow blood vessels stops the throbbing of overstretched arteries.

Depressants

Depressants slow down the nervous system. Some depressants make you feel relaxed. Others, sometimes called sedatives, make you drowsy or put you to sleep.
• Doctors sometimes prescribe another depressant known as a tranquilizer to relieve tension and anxiety. Moderate psychological and physical dependence can result from the regular use of tranquilizers.
• Barbiturates, used in many sleeping pills, cause drowsiness and bring on sleep. They're easily abused. Nervous-ness, loss of muscle control, confusion, and slurred speech are symptoms of barbiturate abuse. Repeated use of barbiturates can cause severe psychological dependence.
• Narcotics numb the senses and block pain.
• Alcohol, another commonly used depressant, should never be taken at the same time as either tranquilizers or barbiturates. The combination of the two depressants can cause unconsciousness and even death.

Vascular Headache: Cluster Headaches

A typical cluster headaches sufferer is a male between ages 20 and 50 who drinks and smokes moderately.

Like common and classic migraine headaches, cluster headaches involve the irritation and expansion of blood vessels. Cluster headaches are so called because the extremely painful attacks associated with them come in clusters or groups. Despite experts' disagreement about naming the disorder, sufferers describe the headache in the same way—almost unbearable. Victims cry out in pain, pace up and down, sometimes lose control of themselves in their efforts to stop the pain, and cannot sit still. Because of the severe pain, some sufferers attempt suicide during an attack.

The disorder is cyclic; that is, the headaches recur in patterns, though the patterns may vary from person to person. One victim may have 30-minute headaches three or four times a day for 10 weeks, while another may have 90-minute headaches twice a week for 6 months. Although cluster headaches occur in any season, they're more common in the spring and fall. Usually, the pattern stops abruptly at some point, only to recur later. For some victims, the cluster headaches never return; for others, they almost never go away. A sufferer may have to endure many headaches a day for years.

The words "burning," "stabbing," and "searing" describe cluster headache pain, which usually hits one side of the head. The pain comes with no warning or prodrome and often awakens its victim. Typical symptoms include eye redness and tearing, runny nose, or nasal stuffiness on the side where the headache starts. The pain may then center on the lower or upper cheek, the lower part of the face, or the neck. Occasionally, the pain will spread to the other side of the head and neck as well.

Who gets cluster headaches

People don't inherit the susceptibility to cluster headaches as they do with migraines. Cluster headache experts disagree about the personality of the cluster headache sufferer, but they agree on two facts: those with cluster headaches drink and smoke moderately,

Cluster headache clues

If you have one or more of these symptoms, you may have cluster headaches.

- *Your headaches are excruciatingly painful and last for 30 to 60 minutes.*
- *One eye tears, and your nose is stuffy or runny on the same side as the pain.*
- *Drinking brings on the headache.*
- *Your headache attacks occur in clusters of about 4 to 6 in 1 day.*

Case study: Cluster headaches

Dennis Ramirez, age 47, and his wife Lena have been happily married for 25 years. Their two children are 2nd- and 4th-year college students.

Dennis's headaches started during a happy time—just before Thanksgiving, with the family celebrating his son's acceptance into medical school.

During the celebration, Dennis suddenly clutched his right temple and began pacing in great pain. He said the pain felt like a poker piercing his eye. His right nostril was stuffy at the same time that his right eye was tearing. Dennis experienced five similar headache episodes a day for several days after the party.

Dennis's family doctor gave him a thorough physical and sent him for some neurologic tests. Dennis had suffered cluster headaches.

and over 90% are males between the ages of 20 and 50.

Since cluster headaches are vascular headaches, substances that enlarge blood vessels may provoke them. The best known trigger is alcohol. Ingesting nitrite-containing meats, nitroglycerin for heart failure, and histamines can also provoke a cluster headache, as can sudden temperature changes.

Treatment

—Seek medical attention. You won't need much encouragement to seek help because of the pain's intensity and frequency.

—You won't find aspirin or aspirin substitute much help because its action time is too slow.

—During cluster headache attacks, don't drink alcohol or smoke tobacco.

Medication

—During the attack, your doctor may administer oxygen for 15 minutes. The oxygen hinders the pro-

How your body absorbs drugs

Before any drug can relieve your headache, your body must absorb it—get the drug into the bloodstream. How the drug enters your body helps determine how fast it can bring relief.

For instance, if the doctor gives you a drug intravenously—through a needle directly into a vein—you have 100% of the drug in your bloodstream right away. If he gives you a shot in a muscle, your body must absorb the drug through the muscle first, another relatively fast process.

Drugs in other forms usually take longer to absorb. A rectal suppository, nasal spray, or oral drug (a drug that you take by mouth) must be absorbed through the membranes that line the rectum, nose, or stomach. Rather slowly, the drug passes through cells in these areas to the bloodstream. In many cases, an oral drug brings the slowest relief, because so many things can affect the stomach and other parts of the digestive tract. Food, fluids, and antacids in the stomach can affect drug absorption. So can the condition and acidity of the digestive tract and the speed of the blood flow to it.

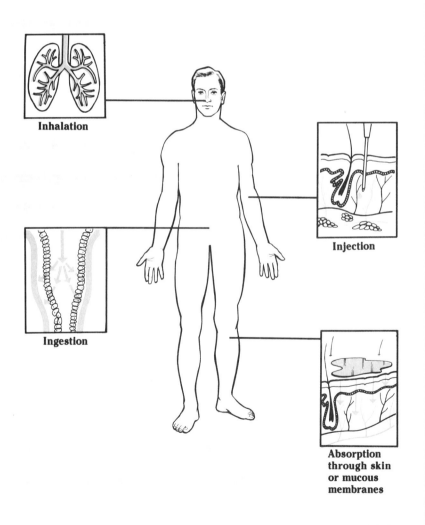

Inhalation

Injection

Ingestion

Absorption through skin or mucous membranes

Thermograms

Thermography measures surface heat. A normal thermogram displays a symmetrical pattern with slight temperature variations. Thermograms of cluster headache patients show cool spots during a cluster attack. These cool spots represent reduced circulation.

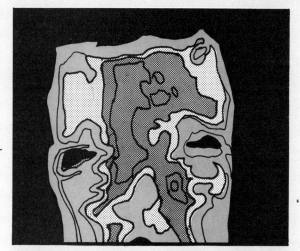

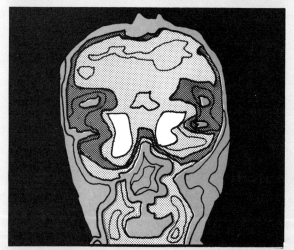

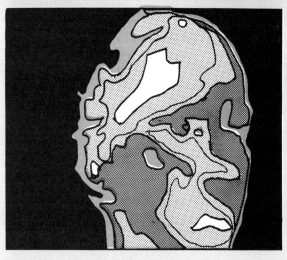

duction of a prostaglandin that causes blood vessel enlargement. He may also give you an injection of dihydroergotamine mesylate.

—Ergotamine as an inhalant or a rectal suppository will reach your blood vessels rapidly.

—If your attacks don't respond to these medications, your doctor may prescribe steroids.

Prevention

—Many people benefit from methysergide (Sansert) as a preventive treatment; however, cluster headache patients with vascular disease, high blood pressure, or impaired liver or kidney function should not take methysergide. If you can tolerate the drug, your doctor may prescribe 6 to 12 mg daily for 4 weeks.

—As an alternate treatment, your doctor may prescribe prednisone in 20-mg doses, twice a day for 2 weeks. Prednisone reduces inflammation, but if you use it for long periods, you'll experience side effects, including inflamed and blocked veins (thrombophlebitis), overweight, abnormal hair growth, and stomach ulcers.

—If you can't take methysergide or prednisone, your doctor may prescribe lithium carbonate one to three times a day for 3 to 7 days. Side effects of lithium carbonate include muscle weakness and coordination loss.

—Give up smoking.

—Reduce alcohol intake.

6

Muscle Contraction (Tension) Headaches

Muscle contraction headache usually causes pain in the temples and forehead or in the back of the head and neck.

With the exception of the "sinus headache"— a rarer headache than advertisements would have you believe—most headaches that actors dramatize in ads for aspirin, aspirin substitutes, or aspirin compounds are muscle contraction, or tension, headaches.

Although the severity of muscle contraction headache pain may vary, the pain is usually dull and persistent. Sufferers tend to describe it as a heaviness, pressure, or tightness. "A band or tight cap on the head" and a "weight on top of the head" are two common descriptions. The head pains and other sensations of the muscle contraction headache occur usually in the temples and forehead or in the back of the neck and head. Unlike classic migraines, muscle contraction headaches usually give no warning signs or visual symptoms, and they don't seem to be caused by food or hormonal changes.

What is a muscle contraction headache? Contrary to what its other name, tension headache, would lead you to believe, it's not necessarily a headache associated with emotional tension. (Many nontension headaches are triggered by stress or emotions.) A tension headache involves a muscle contraction or spasm in the head or neck. The muscle contractions represent automatic physical responses to emotional or physical problems.

If you touch your scalp or neck muscles during a muscle contraction headache, you'll feel tight muscles, tender to the touch. If you felt the same pain in your calf muscle, you might think you had a muscle cramp. Although the muscle contraction causes the primary discomfort in a tension headache, the tendons, nerves, and blood vessels within and around the muscles also cause pain.

Two types

The two types of muscle contraction headaches are episodic, the more common one, and chronic. If you're an episodic headache sufferer you probably don't seek medical attention for your headaches because you can usually control them with over-the-counter remedies.

(text continued on page 37)

The pain process in muscle contraction (tension) headache

Muscle-contraction-headache pain begins when a muscle in the scalp, neck, or shoulder tenses or tightens. The contracted muscle squeezes its supplying blood vessels. As a result, the tissues surrounding the tightened muscle don't receive the blood and oxygen they need.

The cells in the tissues continue to work with inadequate oxygen, but they suffer temporary damage. In addition,

they release pain-inducing chemicals, such as bradykinin, histamine, and serotonin, and pain sensitizers such as prostaglandins.

Nearby nerve fibers pick up the chemical and electrical messages and take them to the brain. The pain signals travel to other nerves on the way to the spinal cord and then to the brain. The brain itself does not feel pain, but it interprets the pain and you feel it.

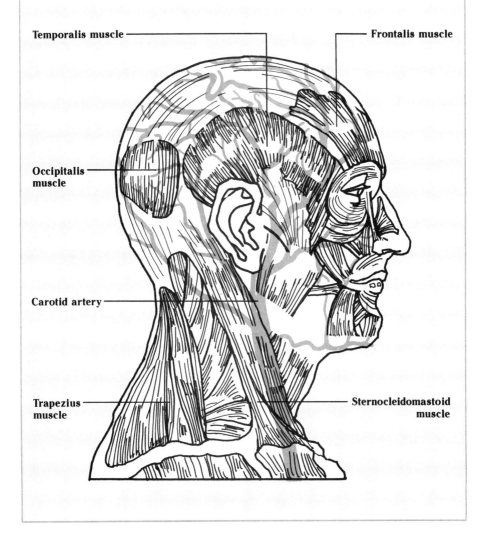

Temporalis muscle

Frontalis muscle

Occipitalis muscle

Carotid artery

Trapezius muscle

Sternocleidomastoid muscle

Case study: Muscle contraction headache

At college, Nicole Claro earns living-expense money typing term papers for other students. In addition to this work, she performs secretarial duties in the English department for 8 hours a week. About 3 months ago, Nicole began experiencing terrible headaches. Until that time, she had been able to control most of her headaches with aspirin. Suddenly, daily aspirin didn't end her headaches—a dull aching pain in the back of her head with knots of tightened neck and shoulder muscles. She didn't wake up with a headache, but she developed one each day. By bedtime she could barely turn her head. Finally, Nicole visited her doctor.

After taking a case history and giving her a physical, the doctor discussed Nicole's headaches. Answering his questions, Nicole realized that in doing her part-time typing and secretarial work, she kept her head and neck in awkward positions for long periods. The doctor explained that the strain on her head and neck was causing muscle contraction headaches.

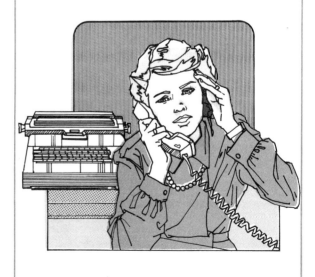

Furthermore, your headaches probably occur infrequently. You probably need not worry about an occasional tension headache, even though it may waste your time, as physical discomforts do.

You should know, however, that serious problems may result from prolonged self-treatment of chronic (occasional) tension headaches. If you have occasional tension headaches but take aspirin just to ward them off, you may be taking risks. First, you need to find the source of recurring headaches. Then, you need to see a doctor so that you can find ways to cope with the headaches, especially if your headache accompanies insomnia, indigestion, or an inability to concentrate.

Who gets muscle contraction headaches

Just about everybody suffers from an occasional tension headache. If you sit at a desk or typewriter all day, if you have to maintain a rigid neck or head posture for long periods, if you're a worried or nervous person with a heavy work schedule, if you can't relax easily, if you're angry or depressed and unable to express or deal with those feelings, you probably suffer tension headaches.

Treatment: Occasional muscle contraction headaches

A simple episodic muscle contraction headache may improve, without any medication, in 5 to 10 minutes with exercise, rest, relaxation, massage, or heat. Choose from these techniques to relieve your symptoms.

—If you can take the time, darken your bedroom, lie down with a pillow under your neck, and close your eyes for 10 minutes. Breathe deeply and concentrate on your breathing.

—Find any quiet place and close your eyes for a few minutes.

—Apply a warm cloth to your head and neck, or take a hot shower.

—Shrug your shoulders several times. Then stretch your neck and head back as far as you can. Make circles with your head and neck. Repeat five times.

—Practice smiling as widely as you can. Use your eyes, eyebrows, the muscles of your cheeks, jaws, and mouth. Hold the smile for five counts and repeat several times. The exercise counteracts frowning, which may cause your headache.

—Have someone massage the back of your neck and upper shoulders.

—If you're wearing contact lenses, remove them. Close your eyes and place the tips of your second, third, and fourth fingers on your closed eyelids. Press gently for 4 seconds. Then, use two fingers to apply pressure to the inner edge of the lower ridge of the eye sockets. Press for 3 seconds and pause.

—Massage your temples. Place the second and third fingers of your left hand on your left temple and the second and third fingers of your right hand on your right temple. Rest your thumbs along the jawbone. Apply slight pressure and move your fingers in a circular motion. (See also "Acupuncture and acupressure," pages 47 to 50.)

Treatment: Muscle-contraction-headache medication

—Aspirin or aspirin substitute should relieve episodic tension headaches. See a doctor if your headache doesn't go away.

—Many doctors prescribe a combination drug like Fiorinal, which combines aspirin and a barbiturate, or Fioricet, which combines acetaminophen and a barbiturate. Other doctors may prescribe Empirin with Codeine, or Tylenol with Codeine. The narcotic analgesic codeine added to a simple analgesic provides extra effect. Take narcotics with care since they're addictive.

—If you experience anxiety or depression with your headache, your doctor may prescribe an antidepressant combined with a mild tranquilizer. The tricyclic antidepressants interfere with your body's use of certain amines, resulting in an increased availability of epinephrine, norepinephrine, and other nerve-stimulating amines. Your doctor may prescribe nortryptiline (Aventyl) or protryptiline daily. If you have a sleep disturbance, your doctor may prescribe doxepin (Sinequan) or amitryptiline (Endep, Elavil) in large nighttime doses. (Warning: A headache sufferer who also has glaucoma, high blood pressure, heart disease, or epilepsy should not take antidepressant drugs.)

—If you have a combined vascular and muscle contraction headache, your doctor may prescribe propranolol (Inderal).

TMJ syndrome headache

Temporomandibular joint (TMJ) problems can lead to headaches. You may have TMJ problems if you:

- *grind your teeth at night*
- *chew with difficulty*
- *feel jaw pain in the morning*

- *hear a clicking sound in your jaw when you chew*
- *have difficulty opening and closing your mouth or moving your jaw from side to side.*

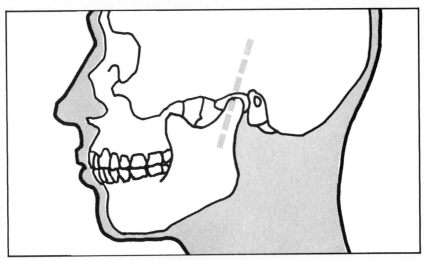

Normal jaw and teeth alignment. Note that the upper and lower teeth mesh.

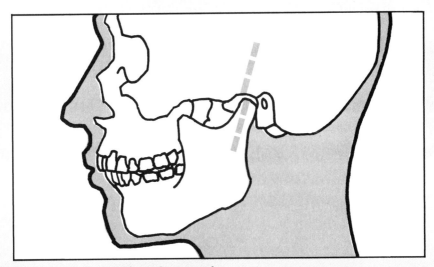

Jaw and teeth align poorly, and upper and lower teeth don't fit together properly, causing TMJ problems.

Head rotation exercises

Repeat these three head ro-
tation exercises five times
each to help treat tension
headaches.

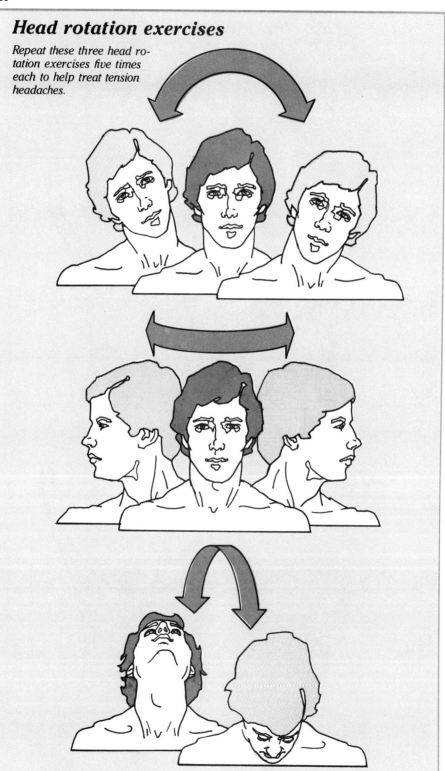

Bone deterioration

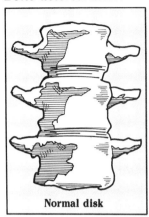

Normal disk

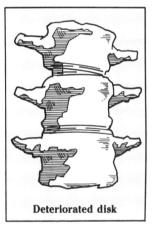

Deteriorated disk

Aging and misuse can result in degeneration and weakening of the disks between vertebrae. When a disk weakens, more wear-and-tear on the vertebrae occurs. One vertebra puts pressure on the next, and the nerve roots and spinal cord can also be compressed. The resulting pain can trigger a muscle contraction (tension) headache.

Muscle-contraction-headache triggers

Once your doctor has diagnosed your tension headache, you'll need to track down the headache triggers. A little self-examination and detective work may help you uncover important clues about yourself.

Posture. The way you hold your head and neck for long periods may be a headache trigger. If you do any of the following activities, you probably hold your head and neck awkwardly:
—type in a chair that's too low
—read in bed while leaning on your hand and elbow
—have long phone conversations with the telephone receiver propped on your shoulder
—drive the car for a long time at night or in bad weather
—paint a ceiling
—watch TV in bed with your chin on your chest or with your head propped on your hand
—slouch in chairs.

Holding your head and neck awkwardly for a long time strains muscles and causes muscle tension. The muscle strain sets off a chain reaction that ends with a tension headache.

Every facial expression involves complex activity of about 30 muscles. Squinting, frowning—even smiling—for prolonged periods can cause muscle pain that triggers a headache.

Disease, trauma, and other disorders. Any of these physical problems sets you up for tension headaches:
—Osteoarthritis, or bone degeneration of the cervical spine (neck), increases your chances of getting muscle contraction headaches. All men and women over age 45 suffer some degree of bone degeneration. As spinal bones become more porous or suffer wear and tear, they can press on nerves and cause pain. When the neck's nerves are pressed, the resulting pain can trigger a muscle contraction headache.
—Birth deformities that involve the neck and spine, as well as injuries such as whiplash, can trigger a muscle contraction headache.
—Although doctors and dentists don't agree on the number of headaches that might be caused by jaw misalignment or temporomandibular joint (TMJ)

Physical signs of stress

- *muscle tension*
- *frowning*
- *headache*
- *clenched fists*
- *rapid heartbeat*
- *awkward head and neck posture*
- *insomnia*
- *restlessness*
- *chronic depression*
- *frequent fatigue*
- *shortness of breath*
- *excessive sleeping.*

problem, neither profession denies that the jaw muscle can undergo strain when the upper and lower teeth don't mesh properly. The misalignment can trigger a muscle contraction headache.

—Although tumors of the upper spine aren't common, they can trigger muscle contraction headaches.

—Imbalance of the eye muscles and farsightedness can create an aching feeling around the eyes. The ache can trigger a headache that may, in turn, spread to the back of the head and neck. Nearsightedness, however, rarely produces headaches.

Poor lighting, precise work performed close to the eyes for long periods, and activities that require repeated up and down movement and refocusing of the eyes may also lead to a muscle contraction headache.

Emotional stress. Emotional stress triggers most chronic muscle contraction headaches. Feelings of helplessness or lack of control, repressed anger and hostility, fear and anxiety, conflict with others, fear of failure, and frustration may trigger headaches in those prone to them. Sometimes these stresses also

Understanding farsightedness

In a normal eye, the cornea and the lens work together to bend light rays reflected from an object and focus them on the retina. Under normal circumstances, the focused rays form a clear image.

In a farsighted eye, the cornea and the lens focus the images of distant objects behind the retina. This, too, causes blurred vision. If you're farsighted and perform close work, or are constantly refocusing to adjust from near to far distances, you may experience a muscle contraction headache.

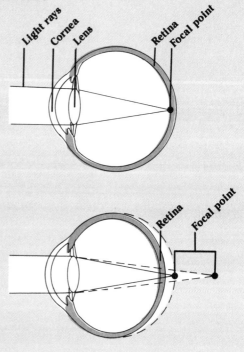

lead to depression, sleep disturbance, weight loss, withdrawal, or excessive fatigue.

When you respond to emotional stress with a muscle contraction headache, you have a physical ailment that's as real as someone else's stomach ulcer provoked by a stressful job or domestic difficulty. Naturally enough, your first concern will be to treat the physical pain, but you'll also need to learn how to prevent future episodes. To start a prevention program, you must find out why you overreact to the stress that triggers your headaches, and you must learn how to cope with the stress. Treatment and prevention always go hand-in-hand.

Prevention: Muscle contraction headaches. Use these eight basic techniques to prevent tension headaches:

—Since overreaction to emotional stress triggers many tension headaches, psychotherapy and psychological counseling rank very high as methods for tension headache prevention. In many instances, you won't find tracking down the headache trigger a simple matter. Even if you're very insightful, you may miss the subtle connection between the cause and your headache.

—If you don't exercise regularly, start now. Choose a convenient time for daily exercise and stick to it. Either join a gym where you can participate in an exercise class or a sport, or select a balanced exercise program that you can do by yourself. If you plan to exercise by yourself, do some research first. Look for a sensible handbook that will tell you how to evaluate your capabilities for a particular sport or exercise program.

—Learn how to relax. Investigate meditation, self-hypnosis, or yoga.

—When you choose chairs, sofas, pillows, beds, and household and office furniture and equipment, take into account the headache-preventing and headache-producing postures that some of them encourage.

Correct indoor lighting

Remember these key points for lighting a room properly.
- *Have two kinds of light: diffuse and special area light.*
- *Reduce contrast by using shades on lights.*
- *Keep shadows away from the work or viewing area.*
- *Prevent the light source from shining in your eyes.*

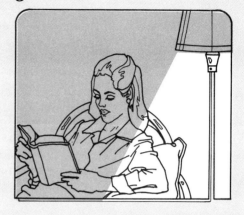

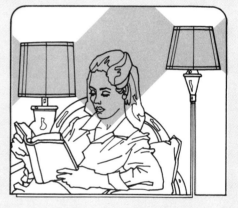

Stress

Stress isn't always harmful. You may feel energized rather than overwhelmed by external pressure and may use stress to motivate yourself and others. Stress can be life-enhancing.

Stress harms you when you overreact to it and suffer physical consequences as well. Since stress is so much a part of everyday life, learn how to respond positively to it.

Chairs with armrests, for example, relieve tension on your neck and upper back muscles by supporting arm weight. Firm mattresses are good for back support. Overstuffed pillows, on the other hand, place your head and neck in an awkward relationship to the upper back. An all-purpose straight-back chair is not the answer if you do a lot of typing.

—Take brief but frequent stretch breaks during activities that position your neck, upper back, and head awkwardly.

—Try to maintain a regular and unhurried schedule.

—Your doctor may prescribe 20 to 40 mg of propranonolol (Inderal) daily, if you get combination migraine–muscle contraction headaches.

—Although antidepressants can be addictive and are never a cure, your doctor may prescribe them when your headaches result from severe depression. As you take antidepressants, simultaneously explore new ways to cope with emotional stress.

7

Supportive Therapies

While therapies such as acupuncture and meditation may not be in the mainstream of modern medicine, your doctor may suggest that you explore nonmedical therapy for your headaches *after* you've had a medical evaluation. If you're a chronic headache sufferer, you may find the formal relaxation techniques of some alternate methods very useful. Don't use these methods as a substitute for medical attention when you need it.

Biofeedback

With biofeedback, you can learn to control some of your body's involuntary functions. At first, you'll use

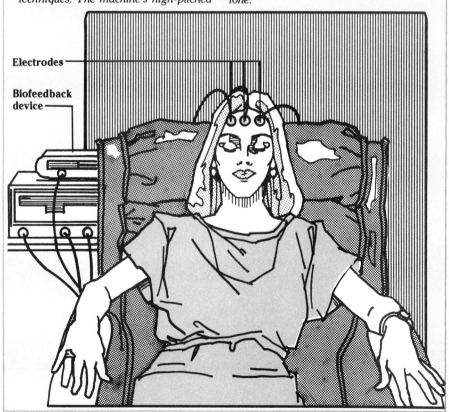

Using biofeedback for pain control

During a biofeedback session, the patient is taught progressive relaxation techniques. The machine's high-pitched warning tone tells her when she's tense. Her goal is to eliminate the warning tone.

Electrodes

Biofeedback device

East meets West

Although many Eastern cultures have for centuries considered the attainment of self-awareness an important goal, Western cultures have only recently begun to pay attention to the disciplines required for such awareness. Biofeedback training combines aspects of modern psychology and electronic technology with some aspects of the ancient Eastern practices of yoga, Zen, and transcendental meditation.

mechanical or electronic devices that monitor, record, and report on your heart rate, blood pressure, and temperature. Your goal is to learn to control these usually involuntary functions.

One of the most successful medical uses of biofeedback training is headache management. Although migraines and tension headaches may have different symptoms, causes, and triggers, most headache sufferers have one thing in common: they exhibit overstated responses to stress and other psychological and physical conditions.

If, for example, you suffer muscle contraction headaches that involve your neck, part of your biofeedback would come from electromyograph (EMG) sensors taped over your neck muscles. Electrodes would feed information from your neck to a monitor. The monitor, in turn, would give you a signal—a hum, a beep, a light—to let you know when your muscles were relaxing. (Initially, the trainer might show you how you are tensing your muscles.) The more relaxed you became, the greater the rewarding signal would be. At first, the trainer might program the machine to register positively when you relax even slightly. Later on, he'd adjust the monitor to respond positively only when you decrease your muscle tension greatly.

Artery changes

Both migraine and muscle contraction headaches involve vascular changes in the neck and head arteries. The tension in a muscle contraction headache compresses and narrows blood vessels, thereby altering the blood flow to the head. The migraine headache sufferer begins with narrowed vessels but develops enlarged vessels during the headache itself. Since a migraine sufferer has unusually cold hands because the body is attempting to keep blood in the brain, he can reduce head pressure from extra blood flow by concentrating on increasing the blood flow to the hands.

Skin temperature biofeedback can help the migraine sufferer increase the temperature of the hands, thus enabling him to abort a migraine in its early stages. In skin temperature biofeedback, temperature measurers are attached to the person's finger. The

How acupuncture works

Acupuncture is based on the belief that disease results from an imbalance or incorrect flow of the body's life force. To restore harmony, the practitioner inserts long, thin needles along a series of meridians, or channels, that affect the aching or diseased body part.

Western researchers have several explanations for acupuncture's success. According to one explanation, acupuncture stimulates the nerve fibers that carry non-pain impulses. These impulses shut the "pain gate" by stopping pain conduction at the spine—before the message reaches the brain.

Another explanation maintains that acupuncture stimulates the body to produce its own painkillers (internal opiates). Enkephalin (produced in the brain) and endorphin (produced in the pituitary gland) act against headaches when released into the system. Pain and such types of stress as strenuous, prolonged exercise can stimulate the release of enkephalin and endorphin. The fact that Narcan, a drug that interferes with narcotic action, also reverses the pain-relieving effects of acupuncture indicates a connection between acupuncture and the body's internal painkillers.

person then concentrates on raising the temperature of the hands, and the machine monitors the results. This method seems to prevent or stop migraine and muscle contraction headaches.

A typical biofeedback training program at a local training center consists of two sessions a week for 4 to 5 weeks. You learn to relax the tight muscles of your neck and head, decrease your blood pressure, and warm your hands. During the training period, you can practice at home and keep records of your progress if the training center lends equipment for home use. After the 4-week period, your trainer evaluates the effectiveness of biofeedback for you.

Your doctor should help in the choice of biofeedback after he diagnoses your headaches. Biofeedback is useful for selected headache patients, but it should be only part of a broader treatment. If you suffer classic migraine with warning symptoms, you'll find the temperature training especially helpful. In addition to helping muscle contraction headache, EMG feedback also helps vascular headache because it enables you to decrease both the severity and duration of the attack. If you have a mixed headache (a combination vascular and muscle contraction headache), both the temperature and EMG training will help.

Acupuncture and acupressure

Pain researchers constantly search for new methods to control chronic pain, including headaches. One important nondrug pain-relief technique that remains controversial is the ancient Chinese art of acupuncture. Some pain experts claim that acupuncture can relieve and even prevent pain.

Because acupuncture involves skin penetration, nerve or blood vessel damage and infection are possible. Therefore, United States licensing requirements remain stricter for acupuncture than they are for acupressure and chiropractic. In some states, the acupuncturist must be a licensed doctor.

During a typical treatment, the acupuncturist inserts 10 or 15 long, fine needles at different angles and depths in predetermined spots on the body that correspond to the problem. Then, he twists and vibrates them to increase stimulation. The patient may describe the sensations as stinging, aching, throbbing, or dull pinpricks. Some patients experience light-

(text continued on page 50)

Acupressure

Pressing out the pain

In Shiatsu acupressure, finger pressure is applied to certain sites to relieve pain. To practice how hard to press, use a bathroom scale as shown at right.

Remember to press each point for 10 seconds, and then suddenly release the pressure.

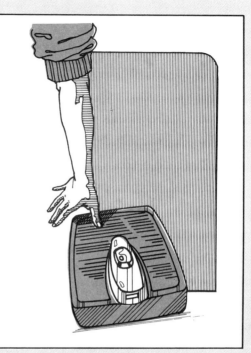

Acupressure exercise for the side of the neck

Press with your right thumb on the right side of your neck and your left thumb on the left side of your neck, applying 10-pound pressure to each of the four points.

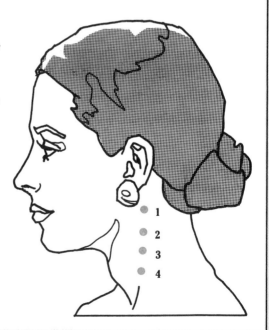

Back of the head acupressure

Use the tip of your index finger to apply 12-pound pressure to the six pressure points on the back of your head.

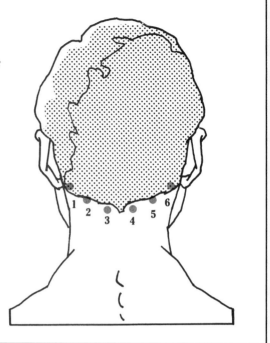

Neck acupressure

1. Lock your fingers behind your neck with your thumbs extending downward.
2. Apply 12-pound pressure to each of the six pairs of pressure points. Work downward in parallel pairs.

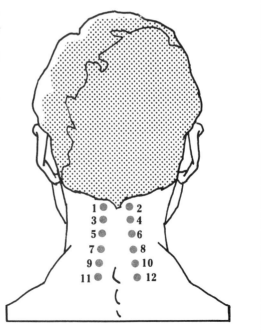

Chiropractic

The American Medical Association does not recognize chiropractic as a valid medical art; however, people turn to chiropractic frequently. According to chiropractic theory, pain and illness result from misalignment of the vertebrae. Chiropractors claim to relieve pain and cure disease by physical manipulation of the muscles and bones of the spinal column. If you plan to see a chiropractor, have a doctor examine you first to rule out spinal conditions that could get worse with physical manipulation.

headedness. Some get relief from headache, muscle and bone pain, stress and tension, insomnia, and dental pain after one 20-minute session, while others require 10 to 20 treatments. One of the drawbacks to acupuncture for chronic pain is expense. Furthermore, the condition may require many treatments and provide no pain relief between sessions.

Shiatsu acupressure, an ancient Japanese healing art, involves the application of finger pressure to the body's pressure points to relieve pain.

Before you try shiatsu acupressure, use a bathroom scale to practice measuring 10 pounds of thumb pressure. When you apply pressure, hold the position firmly for 10 seconds, then release it suddenly. Too much pressure is dangerous, but too little is useless.

Massage

Gentle massage of aching neck, head, and shoulder muscles can ease the pain of muscle contraction headaches by warming the muscles and relaxing them. You can also relieve neck spasms and neuralgia with massage techniques.

To find a qualified masseur or masseuse, you should ask your doctor. If he can't recommend one, perhaps he'll suggest some simple massage techniques.

Meditation, yoga, and relaxation techniques

If you suffer chronic stress-related tension headaches, learning how to relax may be an important skill that can alter your everyday life. However, if you're a migraine headache sufferer, meditation won't help you once an attack has begun. It may help to prevent a migraine triggered by emotional stress.

Self-massage

Try self-massage, since you know your muscles and the amount of pressure and kneading they can take. When you use massage techniques, become aware of your breathing, work slowly, try to relax, and don't strain. Before you begin any neck and shoulder massage, relax with neck stretches.

When not to massage
If you have:
- an unhealed fracture
- a cyst or any unfamiliar or undiagnosed mass that you can feel
- severe localized arthritis
- torn muscles
- bone or muscle disease.

Facial massage
Squinting and frowning for prolonged periods can trigger muscle contraction headaches. Facial massage can prevent or ease the headache.
1. Use your fingers to manipulate the tissue under the skin surface.
2. Begin at the center of your forehead by applying pressure with both hands. Manipulate the muscles and move your hands toward the temples and sides of your face.

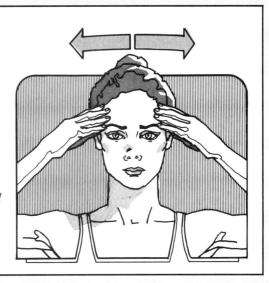

Neck stretches
1. Keep your shoulders stationary.
2. Slowly drop your head back until your chin is up.
3. Slowly stretch your head to the right side, bringing your right ear as near to your right shoulder as you can.
4. As you move your head to the left, try to touch your chin to your chest.
5. Then bring your left ear as near to your left shoulder as you can.
6. Move your head back to the center position, and repeat the stretch.

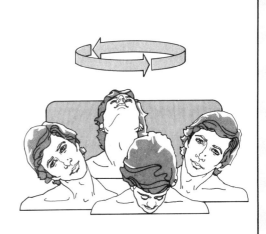

(Continued)

Self-massage (continued)

Kneading

Use this exercise to stimulate circulation and stretch contracted muscle fibers.
1. Lie on your back or sit with your head tilted slightly back.
2. With your palm and four fingers opposing, knead the muscles at the back of the neck by gently pulling the muscles away from the bone.
3. Slowly let go of the skin.
4. Perform the same kneading movement down the back of the neck and along the left shoulder muscles.
5. Repeat the movement along the right shoulder muscles.

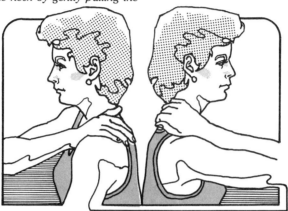

Stroking exercises

1. Sit in a comfortable chair.
2. Close your eyes. Using both hands, place the fingertips of your first, second, and third fingers in the middle of your forehead.
3. Using very slight pressure, slowly move your fingers outward toward your temples with your right hand moving to the right and your left hand moving to the left.
4. After 10 slow strokes, move your fingers back toward the center of your forehead.
5. Then place one hand above the other, and stroke upward.
6. Repeat at least 10 times.

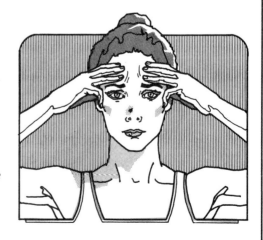

Breathing exercise

Deep breathing not only helps your heart and lungs function more effectively, but also helps you to relax.

You can do deep breathing exercises almost anywhere in any position: sitting at your desk, lying in bed, standing in line at the bus station, or watching television.

Close your mouth and slowly inhale through your nose to a slow count from 1 to 5. As you inhale, focus on moving the air all the way down into your stomach. Let your stomach move out as you fill your lungs. Then, slowly exhale through your nose to a slow count from 1 to 10. Expel all the air you can, moving your stomach in until it feels tight.

As you do this exercise, focus on nothing but the breathing. Try to repeat the procedure at least six times. Try to do the entire exercise at least twice a day.

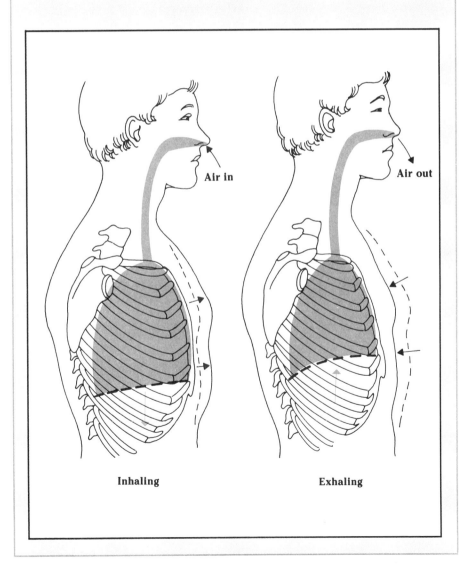

Air in

Air out

Inhaling

Exhaling

8 Secondary Headaches

Headaches can accompany head injuries and many diseases; they're also commonly associated with such symptoms as fever, muscular aches, malaise, and dizziness. Headaches that result from other medical conditions are called secondary headaches. Some secondary headaches signal relatively harmless medical problems, whereas others warn of serious and possibly life-threatening disorders. The intensity of a secondary headache doesn't necessarily tell you the severity of the medical problem. For example, some brain tumor victims experience only slight headaches at a late stage of the tumor development, whereas someone with a relatively harmless sinus infection can have extremely painful, almost incapacitating secondary headaches.

Two main causes

Secondary headaches generally can be classified according to two pain causes, inflammation and traction. Injury, irritation, and infection of pain-sensitive tissue within the skull (intracranial) cause inflammatory headache pain. The different inflammation headaches are named after the primary structure involved. For example, an inflammation headache caused by inflamed temporal arteries is called temporal arteritis. Traction headache pain results from pulled or displaced intracranial tissue and blood vessels, caused by tumor growth or other space-occupying lesions.

Secondary headaches also involve some of the same pain-causing mechanisms as do migraine and muscle contraction headaches. For example, secondary headaches associated with fever, infection, epileptic seizure, hangover, the ingestion of toxic substances, blood pressure changes, or the inhalation of noxious fumes involve widening of arteries within the skull. Secondary headaches associated with arthritic degeneration of the neck (cervical) vertebrae involve muscle contraction.

Traumatic injuries and growths or lesions, such as localized collections of pus (abscesses), tumors containing blood (hematomas), and tumors within the skull, can produce headaches. The headaches result

Where's the pain?
No matter what type of headache you may have, your brain doesn't feel pain. The nerves and blood vessels in the layers of skin and muscle around the skull and brain do feel pain. The site of the headache pain, however, often doesn't occur at the source of the physical disorder. This phenomenon is called referred pain.

Why pain is referred

Pain can be referred because a single nerve or part of the spinal cord receives or carries information from more than one area. The fifth cranial nerve, for example, carries sensation from many parts of the face, the eyes, the mouth, the sinuses, and the covering of the brain. An infected tooth, therefore, could cause a headache in any area of the head supplied by the same nerve.

from direct pressure by the growth on pain-sensitive nerves and from pulled and displaced tissue within the skull. In addition, growths within the skull commonly bring about a muscle contraction headache.

Inflammation headaches

These headaches are usually caused by irritation, infection, or injury.

Allergies

If you have hay fever or seasonal allergy symptoms—itchy, watery, or swollen eyes, sneezing, stuffy or runny nose, fullness in your ears and head—the mucous membranes of your nose and sinus cavities may become swollen. Your sinuses may not drain, resulting in pressure that can lead to a headache. You may also experience some of the generalized symptoms of seasonal allergies, such as fatigue and lethargy. Allergy headaches are not the same as sinus headaches. An infection causes sinus headache.

Treatment: Allergy headache

Aspirin tablets or an aspirin substitute should relieve a secondary allergy headache. Inflamed sinuses will respond to decongestants.

Temporal arteritis

If you press your fingertips to your temples, you'll feel the pulsing of your temporal arteries. Temporal arteritis, an inflammation of those arteries, is of undetermined cause. Early diagnosis is important because the disorder can lead to blindness from a diminished blood supply to the optic nerve. Temporal arteritis rarely occurs before age 50. (But migraine sufferers in the headache phase of an attack may have inflamed temporal arteries.)

Temporal arteritis consists of a prodromal (pre-headache) period and three main stages. During the prodromal period, the person may suffer fever, weight loss, night sweats, and musculoskeletal pain. A headache initiates the first stage, during which patients describe a boring or drilling pain in one or both temples, more frequent nighttime headaches that interfere with sleep, and headaches that are difficult to get rid of. The pain may extend to the scalp, eyes, jaws, and other parts of the face. Chewing, as well as opening and closing the mouth, may be difficult if the temporomandibular joint is affected. A few weeks after the onset of temporal arteritis, the temporal arteries swell noticeably.

Hay fever complications

Hay fever, essentially a lifelong seasonal condition, is more troublesome than disabling. If you suffer from hay fever, you are unusually susceptible to upper respiratory infections. Infection of the sinuses (sinusitis) is another common hay fever complication.

The second stage involves eye complications, and the third stage involves a wide variety of systemic complications, including blindness, stroke, coronary artery blockage, and blockage of circulation to feet or hands.

Diagnosis and treatment: Temporal arteritis

Blood tests reveal an increased number of white blood cells and anemia. Biopsy of the artery may show signs of blockage. High-powered microscopy may reveal artery narrowing and tissue thickening. A temporal arteriogram will show areas where the vessel is narrowed, areas where the vessel is enlarged, and areas that appear normal. Your doctor may prescribe 60 to 80 mg of the steroid prednisone, with the dosage reduced over a 6- to 8-month period. However, you may be given 5 to 10 mg daily as a maintenance dosage to prevent a relapse.

Dental, ear, and eye disorders

Secondary headaches from dental and ear disorders are rare, but they do occur. An ear infection may result in earache, and some dental problems can precipitate a muscle contraction headache. The ear is often the site of referred pain from other head areas. Some migraine sufferers, for example, complain of ear pain.

Secondary headaches from eye problems are common. Eye irritations, such as corneal abrasion, keratitis, and uveitis, cause increased eye pressure, with severe and sustained localized eye pain. Tumors behind or near the eyes may cause secondary headaches. When the condition is corrected, the headache goes away.

Warning
If you have glaucoma, don't take any drugs without your doctor's approval.

Glaucoma. Every adult should annually see an ophthalmologist (a medical doctor specializing in eye disorders) or an optometrist (a professional who examines eyes for visual disorders and may prescribe glasses or lenses but, depending on the state you live in, may not be able to prescribe medication since he's not a doctor) to have a test for glaucoma, an eye disease that can lead to blindness if untreated. The test involves a painless measuring of eye pressure.

Not everyone who has glaucoma suffers from headache pain caused by the pressure. Those who do suffer glaucoma-related headaches may have pain in

What happens in glaucoma

In a normal eye, fluid travels from the back chamber through a meshwork of tissue to an outflow channel called the canal of Schlemm in the front chamber. The fluid travels from the outflow channel into the venous (vein) circulation.

If the iris comes in contact with the meshwork, it will block the fluid. This blockage increases fluid pressure within the eye. As a result, the nerves don't receive their blood supply. Blindness may result if the blockage isn't repaired.

In acute glaucoma, normal drainage may be obstructed by a sudden elevation of fluid pressure that pushes the iris into the angle of the eye where the iris joins the cornea.

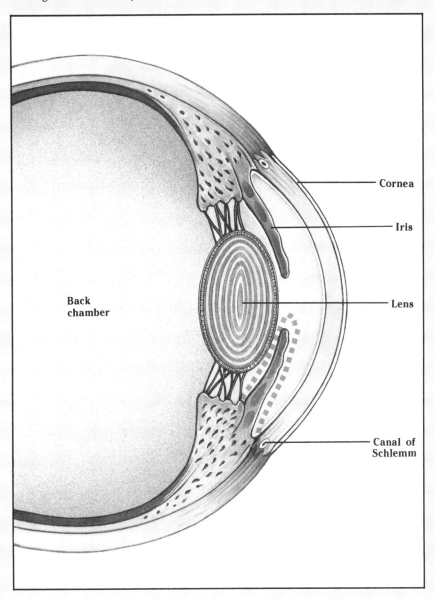

Cornea

Iris

Lens

Back
chamber

Canal of
Schlemm

or around one or both eyes. Other symptoms may include misty or decreased vision; a fixed, semidilated pupil; nausea; and vomiting.

Doctors can treat glaucoma with medication or surgery, depending on the condition's severity. Glaucoma patients should avoid tricyclic antidepressants, antihistamines, some tranquilizers, and drugs for nausea.

Upper respiratory infection

Upper respiratory tract viral or bacterial infection can precipitate a severe headache. In fact, the headaches associated with fever, flu, colds, and other infections may be more troublesome than the basic disorder.

A headache that accompanies fever and infection develops when blood vessels expand as body temperature rises (nature's way of cooling the body) and sensitive tissue becomes inflamed.

Sinus infection. You have four pairs of sinuses: frontal, paranasal, maxillary, and ethmoid. Sensitive mucous membranes line the sinuses. During a sinus infection, tissues become inflamed and painful as the infectious material irritates the mucous membranes, causing pressure. Although the headache pain associated with sinus infection usually starts over the inflamed sinus cavity, it can spread to other parts of the head. Ethmoid sinus infection can produce pain behind the eyes or at the top of the head. In general, a sinus infection headache is achy, dull, and non-throbbing.

Whenever you have a sinus infection, a lasting fever, or a generalized infection, see a doctor. After he diagnoses the condition, he'll prescribe antibiotics and a decongestant, and he may recommend aspirin because of its ability to reduce inflammation and pain.

Meninges infection. The meninges are the three membranes (dura mater, arachnoid, and pia mater) covering the brain. A bacterium or a virus may infect and inflame the meninges, causing meningitis. Some viral infections such as colds can cause viral meningitis. While not serious, viral meningitis may be uncomfortable. The victim will have a severe headache, with pain radiating to the neck, and may experience vertigo, ringing in the ears (tinnitus), sensitivity to light (photophobia), fever, chills, nausea, and vomiting. Doctors don't prescribe antibiotics

Sinus what?
No matter what you have heard on television or read in advertisements, you DO NOT have a sinus headache without a sinus infection. When you think you have a sinus infection, see a doctor.

What causes meningitis
A bacterial or viral infection, meningitis occurs when organisms enter the meninges through the sinuses, the middle ear, the bloodstream, or a penetrating head wound.

The meninges

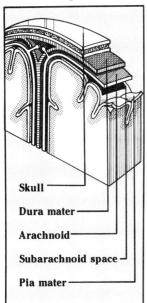

Skull

Dura mater

Arachnoid

Subarachnoid space

Pia mater

The meninges, protective membranes, surround the brain and spinal cord. The outermost and hardest membrane, the dura mater, *is a bone lining. One part of the dura mater extends into the space separating the brain's two hemispheres.*

The pia mater *is the innermost membrane. Between the dura mater and the pia mater lies the* arachnoid *membrane, a thin, weblike structure.*

The subarachnoid space *between the pia mater and the arachnoid membrane is filled with cerebrospinal fluid.*

for viral meningitis, because antibiotics work only against bacteria, not viruses. The body's immune system should be able to fight off the infection, and strong painkillers will help the headache.

Bacterial meningitis, on the other hand, is a life-threatening disorder that begins with a stiff neck and severe headache. Although arthritis of the neck and flu also can cause severe headache and stiff neck, you must consult a doctor if you have these symptoms. Bacterial meningitis requires prompt attention because it can lead to coma and death.

Traction headaches

These headaches are caused by pulled or pushed tissue on blood vessels in the head, usually related to injuries or growths.

Aneurysm

In an aneurysm, an artery wall weakens and balloons (enlarges). The artery may rupture. Doctors don't

Case study: Aneurysm

James Wallace, age 39, knew exactly when his headache problem began. He had received some good news and had run into the house to make a phone call. Suddenly he became dreadfully ill. From "out of the blue," as he described it, he felt a sharp pain in his forehead. The pain soon radiated to the back of his head, and he vomited violently. Nothing like this had ever happened to him. In fact, he rarely suffered headaches. On the following day, the pain was behind his left eye as well.

James didn't have another headache for several months. A second episode occurred as he was lifting a heavy box. He felt a sharp pain in his left temple, and the pain radiated to the back of his neck. Again, he had an episode of violent vomiting.

After the second headache, James visited his doctor. Because of the suddenness and infrequency of the attacks, and the dilation of James's left pupil, the doctor suspected a serious disorder. The neurologic tests confirmed that he had a leaking aneurysm.

Common aneurysm sites

Of the seven types of aneurysms that can occur in the brain, the saccular (berry) types are the most common. The most common sites for berry aneurysms are shown here. Note that most berry aneurysms occur where the vessels divide.

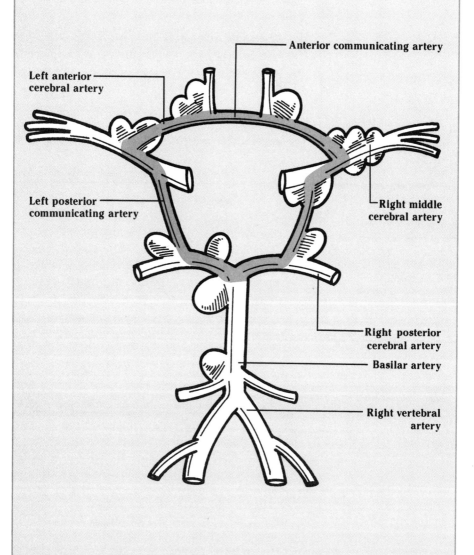

Anterior communicating artery

Left anterior cerebral artery

Left posterior communicating artery

Right middle cerebral artery

Right posterior cerebral artery

Basilar artery

Right vertebral artery

Herniation, or shifting, of the brain

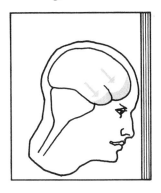

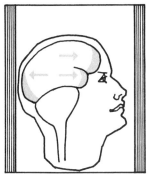

Swelling within the skull or the growth of a tumor or other space-occupying lesion creates pressure within the skull. As a result the brain may shift, or herniate, into the brain stem—which can cause death.

know for certain what causes them or why they rupture. Aneurysms enlarge with increased pressure on the artery walls, and they occur more frequently in patients with high blood pressure. Aneurysms can affect people at birth but usually occur among people in their forties through late sixties.

The rupture of an aneurysm in a brain artery causes a subarachnoid hemorrhage. The blood is released within the skull (intracranially) and can also spill into the brain tissue. The most common initial symptom of a ruptured aneurysm is a sudden, violent headache. (Unruptured aneurysms can cause severe headache near the eyes.) The headache pain may be concentrated in one location or felt generally, and the neck, back, and even the lower limbs may become stiff. Later the pain becomes throbbing and dull. The victim may describe the headache as the most severe he has ever experienced.

Locating the pain at the headache's onset helps determine the bleeding site. The initial headache is due to the enlargement of the blood vessel and the rupture, but the headache changes after the rupture when the tissues covering the brain (the meninges) become irritated by blood.

Other symptoms of ruptured aneurysm include dizziness, vertigo, and loss of consciousness. In a massive hemorrhage, the victim may lapse into a coma.

Brain abscess

In a brain abscess, pus gathers within the brain. An abscess may vary in size from the microscopic to one occupying a major part of one side of the brain. A brain abscess is usually caused by bacteria entering the skull after a head injury or by an infection in the head or elsewhere in the body. Untreated or chronic infections of the middle ear, the sinuses, or the lungs can cause a brain abscess.

Some symptoms of brain abscess include headache, fever, nausea, vomiting, fits (seizures), and stroke-like signs. Approximately one third of brain abscess patients, however, have no fever. An abscess in the part of the brain that controls breathing may cause additional symptoms, such as difficulty swallowing.

Some diagnostic procedures that reveal brain abscesses are skull X-rays, lumbar puncture (spinal tap), and computed tomography (CT) scan. (See page 78.) After a confirmed diagnosis, your doctor can treat the abscess with antibiotics and cortisone to reduce

The stages of a brain abscess

In a brain abscess, pus collects within the brain. An abscess usually develops after a penetrating injury to the brain, after brain surgery, or from a neighbor- *ing infection in the ears, mastoid, or sinus. Patients with a brain abscess are most often between ages 10 and 35.*

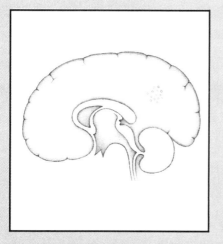

1. An infection spreads to an area of the brain; the site becomes swollen because of an abnormal number of white blood cells.

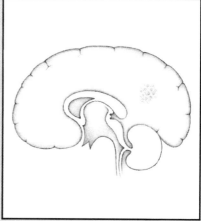

2. The abscess center becomes liquefied dead tissue.

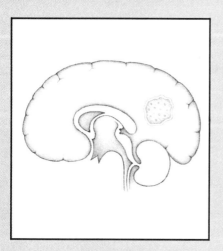

3. A fibrous wall forms around the abscess.

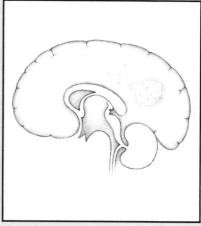

4. Without treatment, the capsule breaks and other abscesses spread to white brain matter and the ventricles. Inflammation of the brain's cover (meningitis) may result.

the brain swelling (cerebral edema). If the abscess continues to enlarge and the symptoms worsen—abnormal slowness of the heart (bradycardia), confusion and stupor, swelling of the optic nerve disk (papilledema)—surgery may be required.

Brain tumors

Headaches are rarely the only symptom of a brain tumor, and those caused by brain tumors are almost always of relatively recent origin. Generally, the symptoms include lack of coordination, altered mental state, weakness, or sensory loss. If you've been having the same type of headache for many years, you probably don't have a brain tumor. If, however, your headaches suddenly change character, you should see a doctor.

The severity of brain tumor headaches varies widely. Generally, as the tumor grows, the pain increases because of pressure on surrounding blood vessels, nerves, and tissues; however, a large tumor may cause no pain while a very small tumor may cause sudden and severe headache, vomiting, and unconsciousness. A secondary headache caused by a brain tumor can be localized to one or both temples or to another part of the head altogether. The pain can last a few minutes or several hours; it can be

Case study: Brain tumor

Louis Suarez, age 68, has been a chronic headache sufferer for many years. According to his wife, he'd been acting differently lately: short-tempered and forgetful, with the problem getting worse.

The family doctor examined Louis and questioned him about his recent headaches. Louis's headaches had changed. The pain he'd been having lately was dull and throbbing. In addition, he complained about sleeping too much and feeling dizzy when he was awake. The doctor noted that Louis walked in an unusual way: he lifted his legs high off the ground.

Louis's symptoms seemed to indicate a serious disorder. His doctor suspected a brain tumor. The neurologic tests and a CT (computed tomography) scan confirmed his suspicions.

Concussion vs. contusion

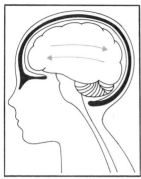

Concussion

Cerebral concussion is a jarring injury of the brain, usually resulting from a direct blow to the head.

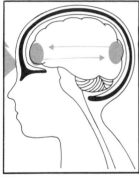

Contusion

Cerebral contusion is a bruising of the brain, usually resulting from a direct blow that shakes the brain. Depending on the force of the injury, small tears in blood vessels, hemorrhages, and brain swelling may result. The contusion victim suffers prolonged loss of consciousness; brain damage may produce temporary or irreversible coma.

constant or intermittent. Usually, the pain isn't throbbing or rhythmic like the pain of a vascular headache, but a brain tumor headache may trigger a vascular headache. In short, a brain tumor headache may manifest itself in different ways. (See *inside front cover* for when to see a doctor for your headaches.)

Meninges tumor. A tumor in the tissues covering the brain (the meninges), or a meningioma, is likely to cause seizures because it compresses the brain from the outside. As the tumor increases in size, the person's vision and intellectual abilities decrease. Headaches are usually a late symptom.

Head trauma

Any mild or severe blow to the head can provoke a headache. Some individuals suffer headaches immediately after an injury; others get delayed but long-lasting headaches; still others experience no headaches even from serious head injuries.

If blood vessels of the scalp and meninges are injured, the person may have migraine and other vascular headaches. The vascular headache may in turn trigger a muscle contraction headache. Treatment for head trauma headaches depends on the nature of the discomfort.

When you've been in a serious accident involving head or neck trauma, see a doctor even if you didn't

Case study: Head trauma

Susan and Chris Rivers were in a head-on collision while driving to a shopping center. Susan hit her head on the windshield and fell unconscious for a short while. When she awoke, she had a throbbing headache, blurred vision, sore neck muscles, and a slight bump on her forehead. She didn't even remember the details of the accident. Susan's X-rays revealed no skull fractures. She did, however, have a concussion, a common occurrence in the type of injury she sustained. Her doctor, concerned about any symptoms that might follow in the next few months, insisted that Susan report anything unusual. Luckily, Susan experienced no further problems from the injury.

have a headache at the time of the injury. You may have injured your spinal cord or neck vertebrae. You may also have a lesion that displays no symptoms.

Intracranial hematoma

Minor head trauma causes most hematomas. The symptoms include headache from the time of the injury and subtle mental changes after 2 to 3 weeks. These changes may take the form of lethargy and loss of initiative. At a later stage, consciousness wanes.

If a hematoma isn't treated, the person's symptoms, including memory loss, confusion, drowsiness, and occasional agitation, worsen. Visual impairment, a late symptom, tends to be less prominent than disturbances of consciousness.

Subdural hematoma
Bleeding between the arachnoid membrane and the dura mater into the subdural space results from a torn blood vessel after a blow to the head, a ruptured aneurysm, or an intracranial hemorrhage.

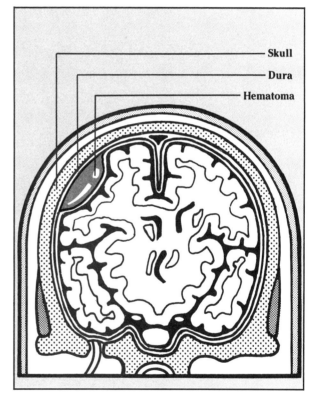

Epidural hematoma

Bleeding between the skull and the dura mater into the epidural space may result from a skull fracture that tears a meningeal blood vessel. Consider an epidural hematoma the most serious complication of a head injury.

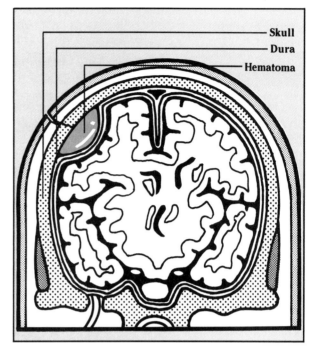

- Skull
- Dura
- Hematoma

Intracerebral hematoma

Bleeding deep within the cerebral hemispheres (intracerebral hematoma) may result from a concussion or a penetrating (knife) injury.

An expanding intracerebral hematoma can cause neurologic symptoms because of decreased blood flow to the brain, increased pressure in the brain, and a shift and distortion of brain tissue.

Small hematomas may disappear on their own. Larger ones, however, must be drained. In some cases, the hematoma can become quite large and spread to both hemispheres of the brain.

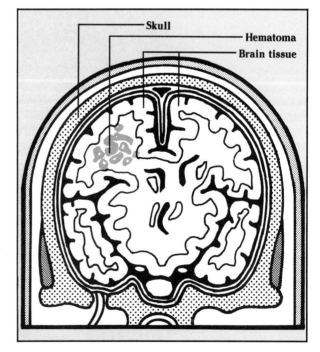

- Skull
- Hematoma
- Brain tissue

Hemorrhagic cerebrovascular accident (CVA)

Bleeding within the subarachnoid space or severe high blood pressure (hypertension) causes hemorrhagic CVA.

A ruptured aneurysm most commonly causes subarachnoid bleeding. The aneurysm, usually located at an arterial junction at the brain's base, ruptures, blood accumulates around the brain, and the victim goes into shock or dies if the bleeding isn't stopped.

Chronic and uncontrolled high blood pressure can also result in cerebrovascular bleeding. A blood vessel, usually an artery, deep within the brain ruptures and causes an intercerebral hemorrhage. With significant bleeding, pressure within the brain increases and brain tissue is displaced or compressed.

Blood pressure and headaches

High blood pressure headaches will go away when blood pressure is controlled with appropriate medication; however, some high blood pressure medications can cause headaches. Since prolonged high blood pressure can damage your blood vessels, your heart, and your kidneys or lead to stroke or heart attack, you should check your blood pressure regularly.

Stroke: Cerebrovascular accident

Cerebrovascular accident (also known as CVA or stroke) can result from changes in the blood flow to the brain from a ruptured blood vessel within the brain or from blood vessel blockage. Blood vessels may rupture from severe high blood pressure (hypertension), balloonlike expansions of arteries (aneurysms), or severe inflammations. Blood vessels can be blocked by plaque (atherosclerosis), or by a collection of fat, blood, or air.

In one type of stroke, a blood vessel, usually an artery deep within the brain, ruptures. Bleeding increases pressure within the skull, and brain tissue can be compressed and die. Coma and death may result. This type of stroke, called a hemorrhagic CVA, is the one most often responsible for a headache.

In the case of hemorrhagic CVA, a waking victim will complain of a sudden and excruciatingly painful headache. Strokes from high blood pressure cause a headache that comes on slowly but develops steadily. Associated symptoms include nausea, vomiting, seizures, elevated temperature, and visual or speech disturbances. If you suspect someone has had a stroke, call an ambulance immediately.

Ischemic stroke. An ischemic stroke results from reduced blood supply to the brain. Blockage of an artery in the brain commonly causes ischemic stroke, which usually occurs in elderly or middle-aged victims with high blood pressure, hardening of the arteries (atherosclerosis), or diabetes. If the victim is conscious, he may have any of a number of symptoms: headache, elevated blood pressure and temperature, stiff neck, vomiting, seizures, slurred speech, numbness around the mouth, or weakness on one or both sides of the body.

High blood pressure (hypertension) headache

Slight to moderately elevated blood pressure rarely causes headaches, but very high blood pressure may cause a severe, generalized pulsating headache. High blood pressure headaches usually occur in the morning and diminish during the day. If you're a migraine sufferer, mild blood pressure elevation may cause a secondary headache—a migraine headache, a muscle contraction headache, or both.

Common sites of hemorrhagic cerebrovascular accident (stroke)

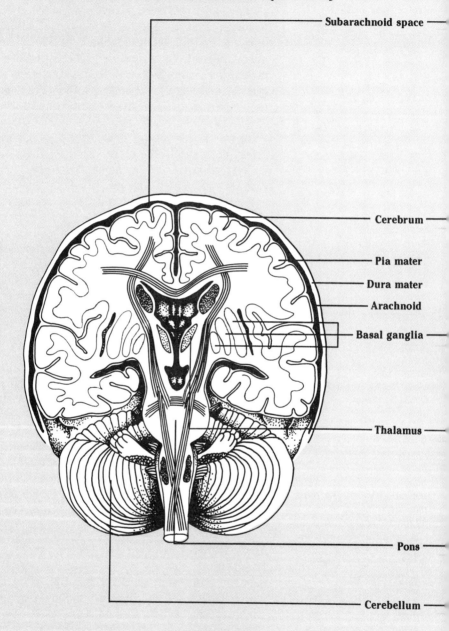

Subarachnoid space

Cerebrum

Pia mater

Dura mater

Arachnoid

Basal ganglia

Thalamus

Pons

Cerebellum

— Sudden and severe headache; possible drooping of the eyelids (ptosis) and enlarged (dilated) pupils; stiff neck; coma, depending on amount of bleeding; nausea; vomiting; seizures; bleeding into brain tissue, causing one-sided paralysis, disturbances in vision, and speech impairment

— Seizures, patient usually not comatose; other findings vary with location—for example, frontal lobe bleeding, causing one-sided paralysis, worse in arm

— Facial drooping; inability to speak (aphasia); paralysis on one side; eyes looking away from weak side; weakness and coma if hematoma expands

— Paralysis or weakness on one side; possible speech impairment and eye disturbance, such as eyes looking downward and unequal pupils that may not react to light

— Coma with total paralysis; small pupils; bloody cerebrospinal fluid

— Repeated vomiting; inability to stand or walk; back of the head headache; dizziness; eyes looking to the side, small pupils; usually no paralysis

Medication

If you're taking medication for an illness and develop a headache, you won't know for certain if your headache was brought on by the medication or by the illness. For example, if you're taking antibiotics for a sinus infection and get a headache, you may have a sinus headache or one brought on by the medication. When you're taking more than one medication, diagnosis becomes even more difficult.

Medications cause headaches by increasing blood pressure, by changing the brain's biochemistry, by causing blood vessels to narrow, or by increasing pressure within the skull.

Medications that contain amphetamine or epinephrine raise blood pressure and can cause headaches. Some drugs prescribed for high blood pressure can bring on headaches as a side effect, and the withdrawal from certain medications like beta blockers (Inderal) and clonidine (Catapres)—drugs used to prevent and abort headaches—can cause increased blood pressure and headaches.

Ergotamine tartrate, the drug used for migraine attacks, can also have adverse effects if taken too frequently. People who take the drug daily may develop a rebound headache when they stop taking it. (See instructions for taking ergotamine on p. 22.) Abuse of ergotamine can cause severe vomiting and circulatory difficulties in the arms and particularly in the legs.

Birth control pills, estrogens, and hormones administered for postmenopausal symptoms can increase the incidence of vascular headaches. If you're a migraine sufferer, taking these drugs may increase the frequency, duration, and severity of your migraines.

Food poisoning

Food containing bacterial toxins can cause food poisoning. When you eat contaminated food, symptoms usually appear within 2 to 4 hours. Symptoms include vomiting, cramps, diarrhea, and sometimes fever and headache. If the attack is unusually severe and persists more than a few hours, call a doctor.

Neuralgias

Neuralgia pain travels along a major nerve pathway. Two neuralgias, glossopharyngeal and trigeminal, are considered secondary headaches. Both derive their

Toxins can cause headaches

If you breathe air polluted by toxins, you can develop a vascular headache. Some toxins, such as those in paint vapors, only cause headaches occasionally. But one toxin—carbon monoxide—commonly causes problems because it's all around us. This colorless, odorless, poisonous gas is a by-product of combustion. You'll find it in automobile exhaust and in the fumes of gas stoves, oil furnaces, open fires, and kerosene space heaters. When it builds up in a room with poor ventilation or outdoors in heavy traffic, it can give people a headache, as well as a fast heartbeat, dizziness, and tightness across the forehead. Here's how:

Once it's inhaled, carbon monoxide binds to the hemoglobin in the blood, preventing it from bringing oxygen to the brain and other parts of the body. To try to get more oxygen to the brain, the arteries in the head enlarge, causing a headache.

Headaches can also result from breathing the fumes of solvents in paints, paint removers, spot removers, brush cleaners, glue, gasoline, and some kinds of foamed insulation. These products cause headaches by forcing the body's nerves to signal the blood vessels to expand. So if you must use them, follow all safety precautions, especially maintaining good ventilation.

names from the cranial nerves involved. (See *The 12 cranial nerves and their tests,* pages 80 to 82.)

Glossopharyngeal neuralgia distributes pain along the glossopharyngeal nerve and the vagus nerve. The nerve path runs along the back of the tongue and throat, the tonsils, the outer ear, and the back of the jaw. Victims claim that coughing, talking, or swallowing can provoke a burning, stabbing, one-sided pain that lasts from a few seconds to several minutes.

Your doctor may prescribe as much as 400 mg a day of the anticonvulsant phenytoin sodium (Dilantin) for the neuralgia. If you can't take Dilantin, he may substitute carbamazepine (Tegretol) with a starting dose of 200 mg that may be increased to 800 mg. Recent studies have shown that the addition of baclofen (Lioresal) to both prescriptions is useful. The average prescribed dosage of baclofen is 10 mg daily, gradually increased to the maximum dosage of 80 mg.

Trigeminal neuralgia, or *tic douloureux*, causes recurrent one-sided facial pain, usually in the elderly. Trigeminal neuralgia rarely occurs before age 50 unless from another underlying problem, and most trigeminal neuralgia sufferers are women.

Trigeminal neuralgia pain travels along the trigeminal nerve, the fifth cranial nerve. In some cases, the lightninglike jabs of pain indicate the presence of an abnormal growth pressing on the nerve. Victims often avoid activities that involve the affected area: washing that part of the face, shaving, brushing their teeth, putting on makeup, or chewing. Trigeminal neuralgia is treated with the same medications given for glossopharyngeal neuralgia.

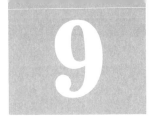

Associative Headaches

An associative headache occurs after you eat certain foods or beverages or perform certain activities. For example, the hangover headache you get after you've had too much alcohol is an associative headache.

Alcohol

Researchers don't fully understand the mechanism of the hangover headache. They do know that the ethyl alcohol in liquor causes the cranial blood vessels to expand, and that the expanding vessels can cause a headache. You don't, however, get a hangover headache when the alcohol level in your bloodstream is at its peak. At the time you experience the hangover headache, the alcohol level in your bloodstream will have dropped considerably and will be almost normal.

The impurities in liquor may cause the headache, or a combination of factors associated with the drinking—the liquor, smoke-filled rooms, perhaps a missed meal, spicy snacks, dehydration (alcohol is a diuretic), loss of sleep, and fatigue—may contribute to it.

Prevention: Hangover headache

—Eat a meal before you go to a party.
—Avoid red wines because they're high in histamines, which expand blood vessels.
—If you must be in a smoke-filled room, try to find a well-ventilated spot.
—Eat only bland snacks when you drink.
—Take a drink with a mixer. Water helps fight the dehydration and reduces the amount of alcohol you actually drink. Fruit juices are good mixers because they're high in fruit sugar.
—If you are very tense, angry, or tired, don't drink.
—The best way to prevent a hangover headache is to avoid drinking.

Treatment: Hangover headache

Hangover headaches are easier to prevent than treat, but try these tips:
—Replace lost fluids by drinking at least 10 ounces of water or juice every hour.

Hangover probability
What you drink (and not just how much) may determine if you develop a hangover headache. The following eight common alcoholic beverages are listed in descending order of headache risk for most people—the riskiest head the list.

Cognac or brandy

Red wine

Rum

Scotch

Beer

White wine

Gin

Vodka

How to prevent a hangover headache

• *Don't drink on an empty stomach.*

• *Choose a drink that's least likely to give you a headache. For most people, the four least likely are beer, white wine, gin, and vodka. (Of course, the last two have a high percentage of alcohol so they may make you drunk faster, even if they don't give you a headache.) Brandy and cognac are the most likely liquors to give you a headache.*

• *Drink slowly so that your body can detoxify what you drink. (Don't have more than one drink an hour.)*

• *Dilute your drinks or have a glass of water after every drink.*

Caffeine in over-the-counter medications

BC Tablets	16 mg
Anacin	32 mg
Cope	32 mg
Midol	32 mg
Vanquish	33 mg
Excedrin	65 mg

—Coffee narrows blood vessels and may be a useful antidote for hangover headache.

—Don't stay in bed. Force yourself to get up at the usual time.

—Take a cold shower or use a cold pack on your head and neck.

Caffeine

Caffeine is a powerful ingredient in many headache remedies because of its ability to shrink or narrow blood vessels. You can help to relieve many headaches by drinking a reasonable amount of coffee; however, you must be careful because coffee consumption in itself can produce a rebound headache.

If you drink 8 to 10 cups of coffee a day, you're probably addicted to caffeine. You may not be aware of the addiction during the work week when you have a cup of coffee on your desk all the time; however, if you spend an active outdoor weekend without your usual coffee, you may get a caffeine withdrawal headache. Excessively expanded arteries cause the headache. (Because of the consistent intake of coffee, these vessels have grown used to the narrowing effects of the caffeine.)

Prevention: Caffeine headache

—Try to limit yourself to two or three cups of coffee a day.

—If you think you're addicted to coffee, don't withdraw suddenly. Cut down gradually by mixing decaffeinated coffee with regular coffee until you can reduce your caffeine intake.

—Check the caffeine content of other beverages you drink and foods you eat. You'll find more caffeine in colas and other products than you might think.

Monosodium glutamate (MSG) headache

MSG acts as a flavor enhancer and tenderizer. It shows up in Chinese and Japanese food, frozen and canned meat, powdered and canned soups, and TV dinners. MSG affects our bodies by expanding blood vessels, which may cause chest pains, headaches, and other symptoms in some people.

If you suffer vascular headaches and can't identify the trigger, check the ingredients on the frozen and canned foods you eat. MSG may be the cause. If you have headaches after meals in Chinese or Japanese restaurants, suspect an MSG reaction. In many Chinese and Japanese restaurants, you can request that the cook not use MSG in your food.

Nitrate and nitrite headache

People who take nitroglycerin tablets for angina, work in factories that use dynamite powder, or consume large quantities of cured meats (ham, sausages, hot dogs) frequently suffer from nitrate headaches. Nitroglycerin, dynamite, and cured meats all contain nitrates and nitrites.

Nitrates and nitrites relax the involuntary muscles. As a result, arteries in your brain may enlarge and bring on a headache. Additional symptoms of nitrate-related headaches include light-headedness, rapid pulse, and facial flushing.

Menstrual headache

For many women, the decline in estrogen during ovulation (around the 14th day of their menstrual cycle) and during the time just before their next period can trigger a migraine attack. Some women who don't suffer from migraines get vascular headaches when their estrogen level drops.

Case study: Hunger headache

Lena Sumner, age 46, decided to go on a strict diet. She was about 15 pounds overweight and felt that part of her problem was her habit of eating every 4 or 5 hours. Her diet regimen consisted of two meals a day—a salad at lunchtime and a well-balanced meal in the evening. She decided to start jogging in the mornings before work.

Lena started to get midmorning headaches during the first week of the diet. The long gaps between meals and the overexertion from jogging contributed to the problem. The changes in her blood sugar level caused the headaches. With the help of a nutritionist, Lena planned a sensible diet and exercise program with very light, more frequent meals and less strenuous exercise.

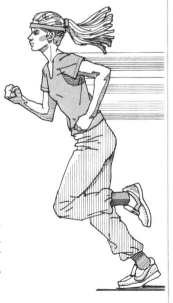

Sex and headache

A persistent headache can obliterate the desire to participate in any physical activity, and sex is no exception. Some people avoid sex because they suffer a severe headache during intercourse, usually during orgasm, with the pain in the back of the head. The headache, called benign orgasmic cephalalgia (head pain), is not a serious condition. On the other hand, headaches during sex can be a warning sign of more serious physical conditions. Avoid self-diagnosis in such matters, and see a doctor for an evaluation if you have this problem.

Weather and headache

Extreme heat or cold—whether from air or water—may cause headaches, especially if you've been overexposed to temperature extremes. If you suffer from a temperature- or weather-related headache, you should follow the remedies on pages 37-38 and 40 for a muscle contraction headache.

Bright sunlight can also bring on headaches. Wearing sunglasses will help you avoid such headaches.

Ice cream headache

When you eat ice cream, sherbet, or any other very cold substance too quickly and get a throbbing pain that radiates from the roof of your mouth throughout your head, you are suffering from an ice cream headache. The sudden temperature change radiating along the glossopharyngeal, vagus, and trigeminal nerves causes the pain. The discomfort doesn't last very long, and you can avoid it if you slowly lower the temperature in your mouth by letting the cold food melt there before you swallow.

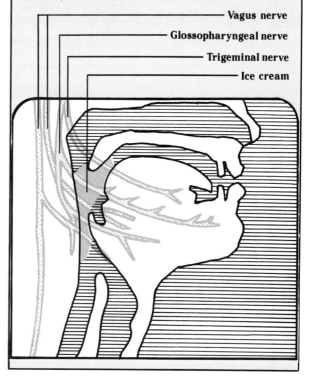

Vagus nerve

Glossopharyngeal nerve

Trigeminal nerve

Ice cream

10

Medical Evaluation of Your Headaches

In addition to checking your physical condition, your doctor will observe your ability to reason, to follow a discussion, and to remember events.

N o matter what prompted you to see a doctor about your headaches, be prepared for a thorough physical examination. Also, be ready to give a detailed medical history of your headaches. If you're seeing a doctor for the first time, he'll want more information about previous illnesses and family history than your family doctor would require.

If you've been keeping a detailed headache diary, you'll be able to give the doctor very useful information. The doctor will ask you to describe the headaches—when they started, the nature of the pain you've been having, how often you've had headaches, and how long they've lasted. He'll want to know if you have any unusual symptoms, such as dizziness, weakness, sensory loss, altered consciousness, or unusual visual symptoms. (See *Symptoms of migraine headaches,* pages 16 and 17, for a more detailed description of these symptoms.) He'll probably ask if you've noticed any correlation between your headaches and certain foods, activities, or a particular emotional experience. He'll also want to know if you've been in any type of accident or if any family member has a history of headaches.

The physical examination

Your doctor will examine your heart and lungs and take a blood pressure reading. He'll probably record your temperature, too. (A fever will alert the doctor to look for infection or systemic disease.) After checking your vital signs, he'll carefully check your head and neck. He'll compare both sides of your face and note any asymmetry of your features, bumps on your head, or bulging of arteries. (If you see the doctor during a migraine episode or a case of temporal arteritis, your temporal arteries will be prominent.)

The doctor will look in your ears and nose for signs of inflammation or infection, and he may check your hearing. He'll closely examine your eyes to check your range of vision, the size of your pupils, the blood vessels, and pressure within the eyes. He may suggest that you have a complete eye examination if you haven't done so recently.

The muscles of your neck, shoulders, and scalp, as

What your doctor will do

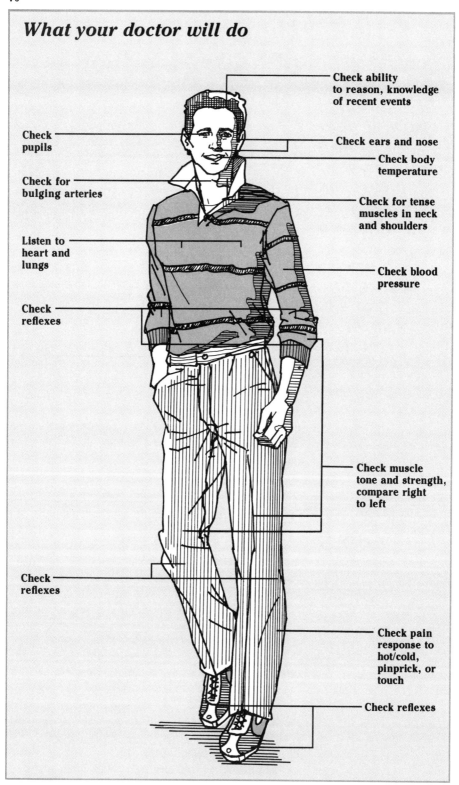

Check ability
to reason, knowledge
of recent events

Check pupils

Check ears and nose

Check body
temperature

Check for
bulging arteries

Check for tense
muscles in neck
and shoulders

Listen to
heart and
lungs

Check blood
pressure

Check
reflexes

Check muscle
tone and strength,
compare right
to left

Check
reflexes

Check pain
response to
hot/cold,
pinprick, or
touch

Check reflexes

well as your neck's range of motion, are also important in the diagnosis. The doctor will look for signs of muscle tenderness and inflammation that could produce a muscle contraction (tension) headache, and he'll note any abnormalities of your neck (cervical) vertebrae. He'll also check the motor functions of your arm and leg muscles, noting significant differences between the left and right side and any peculiarities in your walk.

As the doctor speaks with you throughout the examination, he'll be able to observe some aspects of your mental state, such as your ability to reason, to follow a discussion, and to remember events. He may ask you some questions to check your ability to add numbers or explain ideas. By observing and asking questions, the doctor isn't making a psychiatric profile. Because different parts of your brain perform different mental operations, he's trying to find out if any part needs further investigation.

The doctor may ask you to identify various odors and sensory stimuli, such as a light pinprick, the touch of cloth on your skin, or objects placed in your hands. The sensory tests provide information about how well your nerve endings record sensations.

Very often the doctor's physical examination will give him enough information for a preliminary diagnosis. In some cases, he'll order additional tests to confirm his diagnosis.

Diagnostic and laboratory tests

Your medical history and your doctor's preliminary diagnosis will determine the tests you may undergo. Here are seven important ones.

Angiogram

An angiogram for headache tests is an X-ray of the brain's blood vessels. Angiograms reveal the blood vessel changes caused by tumors, hemorrhages, and aneurysms. The test involves injecting a liquid dye, called a contrast medium, into a vein. During a follow-up X-ray, the contrast medium stands out against other brain tissue.

The test, used when the doctor suspects a serious disorder, causes some discomfort and has some risks.

Computed tomography (CT) scan

CT scanning has revolutionized the diagnosis of brain disorders. A complex X-ray machine rotates around the patient's head and takes slice pictures of the brain at different angles. A computer converts the information into cross-sectional pictures, eliminating the shadows that appear in X-rays. CT scanning enables the doctor to distinguish areas of brain tissues and nerve structures from lesions and other abnormalities.

Although the CT scan involves a small amount of radiation, it's relatively safe technique. It can also be used with a contrast medium to highlight tissue details.

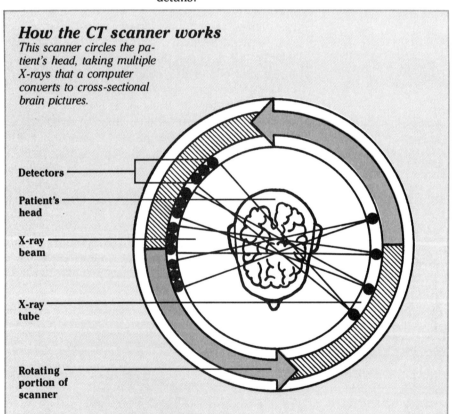

How the CT scanner works

This scanner circles the patient's head, taking multiple X-rays that a computer converts to cross-sectional brain pictures.

Detectors

Patient's head

X-ray beam

X-ray tube

Rotating portion of scanner

Brain scan

During a brain scan, you have a small amount of a radioactive material injected into your bloodstream, and the tissue surrounding the blood vessels absorbs some of it. Abnormal tissue picks up abnormal amounts of the radioactive material. A scanning device measures the results.

How a brain scan works
After the patient receives intravenous injection of a special dye, a technician moves a camera or scanner back and forth to provide images of the brain's blood flow.

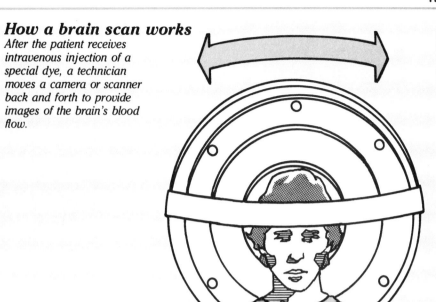

Lumbar puncture (spinal tap)

A lumbar puncture tests cerebrospinal fluid (CSF). The doctor inserts a needle between two vertebrae in the lumbar region of the back. Once the needle enters the space around the spinal cord where the CSF is located, the doctor can measure fluid pressure and remove a fluid sample for analysis. Under normal circumstances, the CSF is clear. Cloudy fluid indicates excessive white blood cells and decreased sugar, signs of an infection. After a subarachnoid hemorrhage (see page 61), the fluid will contain an excessive number of red blood cells and will appear bloody.

(text continued on page 83)

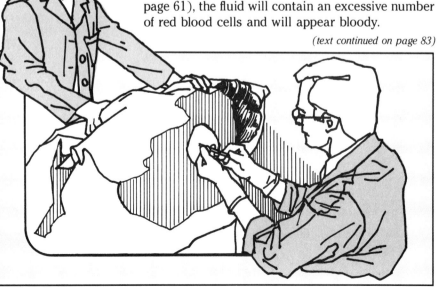

The 12 cranial nerves and their tests

Thorough neurologic examination
includes checking the 12 cranial nerves.

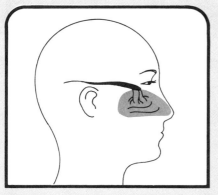

1. Olfactory

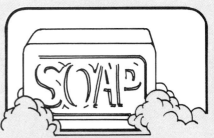

You may be asked to identify the smell
of soap and tobacco.

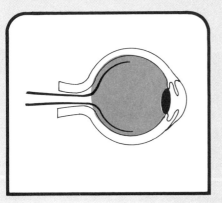

2. Optic

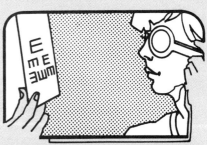

You may be given an eye examination.

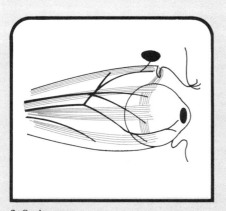

3. Oculomotor
4. Trochlear
6. Abducens

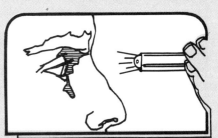

The response of your pupils to light,
your up-and-down gaze, and your side-
to-side gaze may be checked.

81

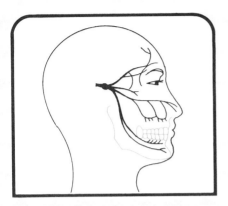

5. Trigeminal

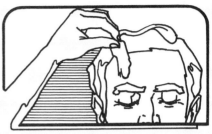

You may be asked to identify a sound or other stimulus to two senses at the same time, and your blink reflex may be checked.

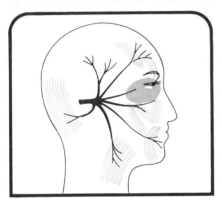

7. Facial

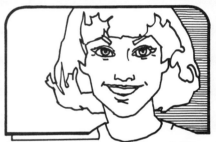

You may be asked to smile or wrinkle your brow.

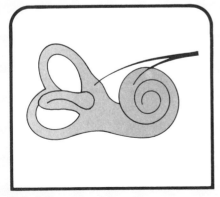

8. Auditory

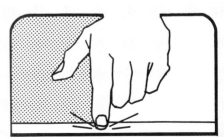

You may be asked to identify the sound of tapping fingertips.

(Continued)

The 12 cranial nerves and their tests (continued)

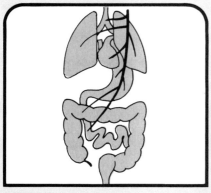

9. Glossopharyngeal
10. Vagus

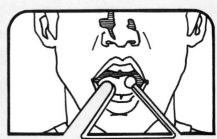

You may have your gag reflex checked.

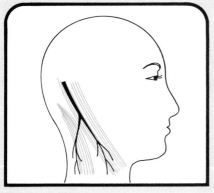

11. Spinal accessory

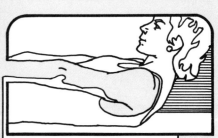

You may be asked to elevate your shoulders.

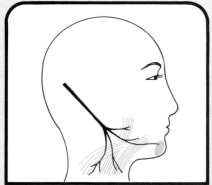

12. Hypoglossal

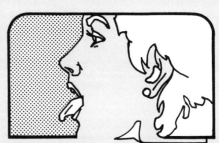

You may be asked to stick out your tongue.

Magnetic resonance imaging (MRI)

MRI, a new and very expensive diagnostic technique, measures radiofrequency signals emitted by cell nuclei. It's an advance over the CT scan, giving both clearer pictures and chemical information about the tissue being studied.

Myelogram

During a myelogram, the doctor first injects a liquid contrast medium directly into the lumbar subarachnoid space. The contrast medium outlines the spinal canal and higher regions if the patient is tilted. The X-ray reveals abnormalities of the spinal column, intervertebral disks, and the brain stem.

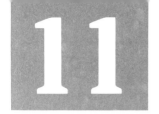

Questions about Headaches

Q. Can you get more than one type of headache at the same time?

A. Yes. One type can serve as a trigger for another. For example, if you have a tendency to get migraine headaches and you overreact to stress, you may trigger a muscle contraction (tension) headache. When you display the symptoms of two headache types, you have what is called a mixed headache.

Q. Can migraines be cured?

A. No. But you can prevent them or use effective medications after one develops.

Q. Is sinus headache very common?

A. No. If you have a sinus infection, you may get a sinus headache, but, in fact, sinus headaches are rarer than advertisements would have you think. Many people who think they have sinus headaches actually have muscle contraction headaches.

Q. Are headache triggers the causes of headaches?

A. No. If you tend to get a particular headache type, a trigger usually sets if off. Muscle contractions in the neck, head, and possibly the shoulders cause a muscle contraction headache. The way you hold your head, cradle a telephone between your chin and shoulder, or overreact to emotional stress may trigger the headache. In the case of migraines, no one has precisely defined the mechanism of a migraine headache, and no one has figured out what causes them; however, researchers have identified the migraine triggers.

Q. Is reaction to stress always a headache trigger?

A. No. Several people may experience the same stressful circumstances, but react differently. One person's reaction to stress may trigger a headache.

Q. Do men get common migraine headaches? Most books and articles on headaches lead you to believe that women are the only victims.

A. Men do get migraines and every other type of headache, but more women than men seek medical attention for headaches, which partly explains the figures in books. Men, however, get more cluster headaches than women do.

Q. What is the difference between a classic and a common migraine?

A. Unlike the common migraine sufferer, the classic migraine sufferer usually experiences an aura, or prodrome—painless warning signs of an oncoming attack.

Q. Who should take medication to prevent migraines?

A. If you get more than one or two migraines a month, your doctor may prescribe preventive medication.

Q. Why does coffee help some headaches and make others worse?

A. Coffee narrows your blood vessels, which may help if your headache is caused by expanded blood vessels. Like any stimulant, however, coffee can be abused. If you drink excessive coffee or other beverages that contain caffeine and take over-the-counter medications that contain caffeine, you can get a toxic reaction to coffee.

Q. Are muscle contraction headaches caused by stress?
A. Stress can trigger a muscle contraction headache, but the headache's cause is muscle contraction.

Q. Can arthritis trigger a headache?
A. Yes. Arthritis of the cervical vertebrae can trigger a muscle contraction headache.

Q. How can psychotherapy and psychological counseling help a headache sufferer?
A. If overreaction to stress triggers your headache, therapy or counseling may change the way you react to stress. If you have chronic pain, the therapy may help you cope with pain.

Q. How can biofeedback training help a headache sufferer?
A. With biofeedback training, you can learn to relax tight muscles and control involuntary body functions, such as blood pressure and circulation.

Q. When should I see a doctor for headaches?

A. You should see a doctor if your headaches:
—assume a chronic pattern and you're not a headache sufferer
—interfere with your life-style
—are associated with pain in a particular organ
—follow a head injury
—don't respond to aspirin or aspirin substitute
—are accompanied by unusual symptoms, such as nausea and vomiting.
In short, don't self-diagnose or self-treat headaches that are more frequent than occasional.

Q. Is extra-strength aspirin better for headache than plain aspirin or aspirin substitute?
A. No. These products are a more expensive way for you to get extra caffeine. Aspirin's anti-inflammatory ability is what helps a headache sufferer.

Q. Does the brain hurt during a headache?
A. No. The brain doesn't feel pain, but it does register pain or transfer a pain message.

Q. What are some of the foods and chemicals in foods that can trigger headaches?
A. Aged cheeses; red wine; hot dogs and cured meats that contain nitrates; alcohol; chocolate, coffee, tea, and other products that contain caffeine; ice cream; and monosodium glutamate (MSG).

Drugs for Headache Relief

The following chart shows you which drugs can prevent and/or provide relief for which headaches, along with each drug's side effects and other special information. If you must take any of these drugs, remember to:
• avoid driving, operating heavy machinery, and mixing alcohol or other depressants with drugs that cause drowsiness
• see your doctor if you have side effects
• see your doctor before taking any drug if you're pregnant.

Migraine headache treatment

Drug	Side effects	Special considerations
dihydroergotamine† (in D.H.E. 45 injection)	*Minor side effects:* tingling in the hands or feet, dizziness, nausea, vomiting, diarrhea, stomach or muscle pains, itching, and thirst *Serious side effects:* chest pain and signs of reduced blood flow, such as abdominal pain and coldness or numbness in the hands and feet	• Talk to your doctor before taking this drug if you have high blood pressure, heart disease, blood vessel disease, peptic ulcers, or liver or kidney disease. • Don't take more than 6 mg in 1 week.
ergotamine† (in Ergomar sublingual tablets, Ergostat sublingual tablets, Wigrettes sublingual tablets, Medihaler Ergotamine aerosol spray, Cafergot and Cafergot P-B tablets or suppositories, and Wigraine tablets)	Same as side effects of dihydroergotamine	• Talk to your doctor before taking this drug if you have high blood pressure, heart disease, blood vessel disease, peptic ulcers, or liver or kidney disease. • Don't take more than 10 mg of sublingual tablets or 15 inhalations of aerosol spray in 1 week.
isometheptene† (in Midrin, which also contains dichloralphenazone and acetaminophen)	*Minor side effects:* dizziness, insomnia or drowsiness, nausea, and vomiting *Serious side effects:* abnormal heartbeat and weakness	• Talk to your doctor before taking this drug if you have high blood pressure, glaucoma, or kidney, liver, or heart disease.
*codeine†, oxycodone†, combination drugs that contain butalbital†, ibuprofen, acetaminophen, and aspirin and other salicylates	*See* Muscle-contraction-headache treatment, *pages 89 to 90.*	*See* Muscle-contraction-headache treatment, *pages 89 to 90.*

*Effective for migraine treatment but principally used for muscle-contraction-headache treatment.
†Available by doctor's prescription only.

Migraine headache prevention

Drug	Side effects	Special considerations
methysergide† (in Sansert)	*Minor side effects:* nausea, vomiting, abdominal cramps, weight gain, and tingling in the hands or feet *Serious side effects:* chest pain, difficulty breathing, painful urination, or kidney pain; signs of reduced blood flow, such as cold or numb hands or feet; hallucinations; and depression	• Talk to your doctor before taking this drug if you have high blood pressure, heart disease, blood vessel disease, peptic ulcers, arthritis, or liver, kidney, or lung disease.
propranolol† (in Inderal)	*Minor side effects:* nausea, diarrhea, dizziness, tiredness, cold hands and feet, and dry mouth *Serious side effects:* signs of low blood pressure, such as persistent dizziness and lightheadedness; confusion; depression; slowed heart rate; difficulty breathing	• Talk to your doctor before taking this drug if you have allergies, asthma, diabetes, emphysema, or liver disease. • Don't stop taking propranolol abruptly because this increases the risk of heart problems.
calcium channel blockers†, including verapamil (in Isoptin and Calan), nifedipine (in Procardia), and nimodipine	*Minor side effects:* dizziness, weakness, nausea, and weight gain *Serious side effects:* signs of low blood pressure, such as persistent dizziness and lightheadedness; shortness of breath; extreme weakness; and ankle or feet swelling	• Talk to your doctor before taking this drug if you have kidney, liver, heart, or blood vessel disease. • Don't stop taking this drug abruptly. • See your doctor if you develop swelling of the feet, ankles, or lower legs.
amitriptyline† (in Elavil and Endep)	*Minor side effects:* drowsiness, dizziness, fatigue, dry mouth, and headache *Serious side effects:* blurred vision, difficult urination, constipation, abnormal heartbeat, fainting, and liver damage	• Talk to your doctor before taking this drug if you have asthma, epilepsy, glaucoma, liver disease, high blood pressure, or heart disease, or if you're recovering from a heart attack.
imipramine† (in Tofranil)	Same as side effects of amitriptyline	Same as special considerations for amitriptyline
clonidine† (in Catapres)	*Minor side effects:* dry mouth and eyes, drowsiness, dizziness, light-headedness, constipation, and nausea *Serious side effects:* depression, nightmares, impotence, cold hands and feet, fluid retention, and weight gain	• Talk to your doctor before taking this drug if you have kidney or heart disease or if you're recovering from a heart attack. • Don't stop taking clonidine abruptly: it can cause increased blood pressure.

(Continued)

†Available by doctor's prescription only.

Migraine headache prevention (continued)

Drug	Side effects	Special considerations
cyproheptadine† (in Periactin)	*Minor side effects:* drowsiness, dizziness, constipation, difficult urination, and dry mouth *Serious side effects:* allergic reactions, such as a rash; confusion; and hallucinations	• Talk to your doctor before taking this drug if you have high blood pressure, glaucoma, thyroid disease, or a urinary obstruction.

Cluster headache treatment

Drug	Side effects	Special considerations
ergotamine and dihydroergotamine	*See* Migraine headache treatment, *page 86.*	*See* Migraine headache treatment, *page 86.*
prednisone† (in Deltasone)	*Minor side effects:* nausea, indigestion, weight gain, insomnia, nervousness, muscle cramps, and menstrual irregularities *Serious side effects:* mental or emotional disturbances; signs of potassium loss, such as persistent muscle cramps or unusual tiredness; signs of stomach bleeding, such as bloody or black, tarry stools; high blood pressure	• Talk to your doctor before taking this drug if you're also taking digoxin or digitoxin or if you have diabetes mellitus, heart disease, fungal infections, peptic ulcers, or tuberculosis. • Take prednisone with food or milk to reduce stomach upset. • Don't stop taking prednisone abruptly because this can cause a withdrawal reaction with fever, weakness, and dangerously low blood pressure.

Cluster headache prevention

Drug	Side effects	Special considerations
methysergide†	*See* Migraine headache prevention, *pages 87 to 88.*	*See* Migraine headache prevention, *pages 87 to 88.*
prednisone†	*See* Cluster headache treatment.	*See* Cluster headache treatment.
lithium† (in Eskalith)	*Minor side effects:* increased thirst and urination, diarrhea, and dry mouth *Serious side effects:* nausea; vomiting; drowsiness; weakness; confusion; tremors; seizures; slurred speech; and signs of thyroid gland dysfunction, such as dry or puffy skin, unusual tiredness, and weight gain	• Talk to your doctor before taking this drug if you have epilepsy, Parkinson's disease, or kidney or heart disease. • Drink at least 2 quarts of water daily. • Avoid strenuous exercise in very hot weather. • Take lithium with food or milk to reduce stomach upset. • Salt, sodium bicarbonate, and diuretics can increase this drug's side effects.

†Available by doctor's prescription only.

Muscle-contraction-headache treatment

Drug	Side effects	Special considerations
aspirin (in Bayer, Ecotrin, and Empirin; and in Anacin, Anacin Maximum Strength, and Synalgos, which also contain caffeine)	*Minor side effects:* stomach upset and ringing in the ears *Serious side effects:* allergic reactions, such as wheezing or chest tightness; slow blood clotting; and signs of stomach bleeding, such as bloody or black, tarry stools	• Talk to your doctor before taking this drug if you have peptic ulcers, liver disease, allergies, asthma, or bleeding disorders or if you must take drugs to prevent blood clots. • Don't take aspirin if it smells like vinegar, because it has decomposed and can irritate your stomach or mouth. • Stop taking aspirin a week before you have surgery.
magnesium salicylate (in Doan's pills), salsalate† (in Disalcid), choline salicylate (in Arthropan), and choline magnesium trisalicylate† (in Trilisate)	Same as side effects of aspirin	Same as special considerations for aspirin
acetaminophen (in Tylenol and Datril; and in Excedrin, Trigesic, Duradyne, and Vanquish, which also contain aspirin and caffeine)	*Minor side effects:* dizziness, diarrhea, and stomach upset *Serious side effects:* liver damage or hepatitis	• Talk to your doctor before taking this drug if you have liver disease. • Liver damage can result from overdose.
butalbital† (in Fiorinal, which also contains aspirin and caffeine; and in Fioricet and Esgic, which also contain acetaminophen and caffeine)	*Minor side effects:* dizziness, drowsiness, and clumsiness *Serious side effects:* difficulty breathing; slow heartbeat; liver damage; and mental changes, such as confusion or excitement	• Talk to your doctor before taking this drug if you have lung or liver disease or porphyria (a metabolic disorder). • Extended use of butalbital may lead to dependence.
ibuprofen (in Motrin†, Nuprin, and Advil)	*Minor side effects:* diarrhea or constipation, nausea, dry mouth, and dizziness *Serious side effects:* ringing in the ears; signs of stomach bleeding, such as bloody or black, tarry stools; signs of excess fluid retention, such as swelling of the legs or feet; abnormal vision; severe skin	• Talk to your doctor before taking this drug if you've had abnormal reactions to aspirin or other salicylates. • Tell the doctor if you develop signs of fluid retention, urinary problems, or bleeding stomach ulcers. • Take ibuprofen with food or milk to reduce stomach upset. *(Continued)*

†Available by doctor's prescription only.

Muscle-contraction-headache treatment *(continued)*

Drug	Side effects	Special considerations
ibuprofen *(continued)*	rash; and signs of kidney or urinary problems, such as painful urination or bloody urine	
codeine† (in Empirin with Codeine, which also contains aspirin; and in Tylenol with Codeine, which also contains acetaminophen)	*Minor side effects:* constipation, appetite loss, stomach upset, skin rash, drowsiness, and dizziness *Serious side effects:* breathing difficulty, slow heartbeat, and fainting	• Talk to your doctor before taking this drug if you have heart, lung, or liver disease. • Extended use of codeine may lead to dependence.
oxycodone† (in Percocet-5 and Tylox, which also contain acetaminophen; and in Percodan, which also contains aspirin)	Same as side effects of codeine	Same as special considerations for codeine
orphenadrine† (in Norgesic and Norgesic Forte)	*Minor side effects:* nausea, dry mouth, drowsiness, and dizziness *Serious side effects:* allergic reactions, such as itching or skin rash; rapid heartbeat; fainting; and confusion	• Talk to your doctor before taking this drug if you have heart disease, glaucoma, ulcers, or intestinal or urinary obstructions.

Trigeminal neuralgia headache treatment

Drug	Side effects	Special considerations
carbamazepine† (in Tegretol)	*Minor side effects:* dizziness, drowsiness, dry mouth, nausea, vomiting, and blurred vision *Serious side effects:* severe skin rash, liver or kidney damage, and confusion	• Talk to your doctor before taking this drug if you have liver or kidney disease or a blood disorder or if you're taking a drug to prevent blood clots.

†Available by doctor's prescription only.

13 Keeping a Headache Diary

Think about your last headache. Do you remember what provoked it, what you ate before the headache, how long it lasted, what the pain was like, and what you did to make it go away? If you're a chronic headache sufferer or if you get different kinds of headaches, you'll find you can't distinguish one headache from another unless you keep a written record of each one.

Use the chart on the following pages to record details about your headaches. Each entry will be a significant detail for your headache diagnosis, treatment, and prevention.

You'll record details in each of these areas:

Day, date, and time

The day of the week and date on which you got your headache may reveal a headache pattern. For example, you may find that your headaches always occur on weekends or holidays. This information may be an important clue in tracking your headache triggers.

Situation or triggers

List what you ate, how you felt, and what you were doing before the headache, whether you had slept too much or too little, and any other possible headache trigger.

Pain location

Describe what part of your head hurt and tell whether the pain moved to another part of your head or from your head to your neck. The pain may be on top of your head, in the temples, over your eyes, or on part of your face or neck.

Pain description

Try to describe the pain. Some terms that may help you include throbbing or pulsing, stabbing or piercing, dull, sharp, tightness or pressure, and tingling.

Severity scale

Rate your headaches on a scale of 1-10: 1-3, slightly annoying; 4-5, moderately distressing; 6-8, very distressing; 9-10, incapacitating or unbearable.

Duration

Record the length of each headache, from the first symptom's appearance to the time the headache went away.

Associated symptoms

Your headache may be accompanied by seemingly unrelated symptoms. In fact, your doctor may find these symptoms significant. If you feel sick to your stomach (nausea) or dizzy or if you have other symptoms, record them.

Action taken

List any medication (including the amount taken), exercises, or headache remedy that seems to relieve your headache.

Response

How soon after you took medication or some other action to relieve your headache did your headache go away? Were there any after-effects?

Headache Diary

Day, time, and date	Situation or trigger	Pain location	Severity scale	

Pain description	Duration	Associated symptoms	Action taken	Response

Index